AUDITORY PERCEPTUAL DISORDERS AND REMEDIATION

Auditory Perceptual Disorders and Remediation

By

BERNICE E. HEASLEY

Former Supervisor, Speech and Hearing Therapy
Stark County School System
Louisville, Ohio

With a Foreword by

KENDALL K. WARD, M.A.
Assistant Professor
Kent State University
Stark Campus
Canton, Ohio

CHARLES C THOMAS • PUBLISHER
Springfield • Illinois • USA

Published and Distributed Throughout the World by

CHARLES C THOMAS • PUBLISHER
Bannerstone House
301-327 East Lawrence Avenue, Springfield, Illinois, U.S.A.

ISBN 0–398–02921–0

Library of Congress Catalog Card Number: 73–10020

With THOMAS BOOKS careful attention is given to all details of manufacturing and design. It is the Publisher's desire to present books that are satisfactory as to their physical qualities and artistic possibilities and appropriate for their particular use. THOMAS BOOKS will be true to those laws of quality that assure a good name and good will.

Library of Congress Cataloging in Publication Data

Heasley, Bernice E
Auditory perceptual disorders and remediation.

1. Communicative disorders in children. 2. Speech therapy. I. Title. [DNLM: 1. Auditory perception—In infancy and childhood. 2. Hearing disorders—Infancy and childhood. 3. Remedial teaching. WV270 H436a 1973]
RJ496.S7H4 617.8′9 73–10020
ISBN 0–398–021–0

Printed in the United States of America

K-8

FOREWORD

PHYSIOLOGISTS generally concede that hearing requires a finely wrought mechanism—the most sophisticated employed in our sensory systems. Sound, before it is detected and made meaningful, travels a curious path. It is initiated by any vibrating object; it passes *through the air* to the ear drum; it is converted into a *series of mechanical movements* in the middle ear; and these movements on reaching the inner ear precipitate *electro-chemical impulses* which are discharged along a neural track to the brain. Interpreting these impulses as noise, speech, music, etc. is the function of the brain. When all four components (outer ear, middle ear, inner ear, and brain) perform properly, information is processed auditorially in an effortless manner. But malfunctions can occur and the resultant message may be too soft, scrambled and distorted, or in the extreme, meaningless.

Professional educators have for years recognized the needs of children with visual perception problems and materials are readily available to assist them. Now we are seeing a renaissance in the study of auditory perception problems; their detection and treatment. This book is the result of the author's investigations in this area and will prove valuable in providing practical therapeutic exercises with a minimum of special materials and equipment.

KENDALL K. WARD

INTRODUCTION

THIS BOOK discusses auditory perceptual problems and remediation. An operant approach should be utilized throughout. That is, desired responses, or approximations thereof, should be rewarded while undesired responses should be ignored or responded to in such a manner that they do not reinforce the listener.

The scope and sequence chart found at the end of Chapter I represents a highly compressed summary of the Auditory Perceptual Program. The author has drawn upon her experiences and observations as a listener; a mother; a speech, hearing and language therapist; and as an educator of preschool hearing impaired children.

While the materials of this book have not been subjected to controlled studies, they have been field tested by speech therapists, teachers, and parents, with varying degrees of success. It is not possible to assess the degree to which maturation may have contributed to the success of individuals who have been provided these lessons. The same, however, may be said of general education. Controlled studies should be a natural outgrowth of practical application of these lessons. Criticism is inevitable and desirable, for it imposes responsibility for further study and improvement upon the critic.

This book, then, is submitted as a foundation upon which the educator may build. It is not considered complete. Perhaps it never will be. I hope not. I earnestly hope that in the near future these materials will become obsolete, for this will mean that more effective means of helping auditorially disabled individuals have been developed. Suggestions for improvement of these materials, based upon practical utilization, will be welcomed.

The reader's attention is directed to materials in the appendix of this book. Based upon the sequential lessons found in this manual, Richard Dickerhoof has developed a series of introductory lesson plans designed for either individual or group work. Periodic tests of functioning are incorporated into the twenty-six lessons. This series could well be adopted as a model in providing early stages of remediation for the auditorially disabled individual.

Eunice Shonk has provided a bibliography of commercially available remediation materials which are pertinent to specific components of auditory perception. This, it seems to me, renders a valuable service to the readers of this book.

Without the assistance and encouragement of numerous persons, this book would never have been written. Joe and Jennybel Millen, gave much practical assistance and direction to this text. Dr. Francis Blair, Robert Briskey, Richard Oriole, Kendall Ward, William C. Healey, and Charles Brand have made suggestions which improved clarity and which more nearly assured that lessons followed a logical sequential order. Nancy Waffler kindly posed for the vowel pictures.

Mary Louise Wilson, who typed this manuscript, also served as a proofreader and as a surrogate conscience during those periods when the author tended to neglect completion of the work. To the Thomas Publishing Company, the author expresses her appreciation for encouragement and enduring patience.

BERNICE E. HEASLEY

CONTENTS

AUDITORY PERCEPTUAL DISORDERS AND REMEDIATION

CHAPTER I

SUGGESTIONS FOR USING THIS BOOK

THE AUDITORY PERCEPTUAL training lessons in this book follow a carefully structured heirarchy. Based upon the developmental model, the lessons are graduated in terms of difficulty, length of lesson, and numbers of processes introduced. This closely approximates the normal sequential landmarks of childhood development in the areas of hearing, speech and language.

Sample lessons are provided following certain sections. These lessons include a checklist to indicate the listener's readiness to progress to the next lesson.

The lessons in this book will serve both to identify the areas in which an individual is experiencing auditory perceptual problems, and also as remediation.

Beginning with Chapter V, the auditory perceptual exercises have three broad bases: remediation utilizing gross sounds, animal sounds as a transition to speech sound, and the sounds of speech.

Although the listener who suffers a problem with auditory perception may already recognize many or all of the gross sounds introduced in these lessons, there is good reason for progressing through this series. It is in keeping with the developmental model and represents a natural starting point. Of even more critical importance, however, is the probability that while recognizing the gross sounds, the listener is unable to process, retreive and identify them in a more involved task. Furthermore, the gross auditory perceptual lessons serve to develop attention, attention span, memory, and other auditory skills in a non-threatening setting. The use, initially of nonspeech materials may be highly important for individuals who are emotionally disturbed or who are aphasic. Speech is a subtle, abstract human skill; one of man's most recent symbolic acquisitions. The responsibility for verbal speech is, for many individuals, highly anxiety provoking.

Finally, working through the gross and environmental sound exercises provides the teacher an opportunity to develop a way of teaching. It provides the listener a way of responding to the training tasks. This becomes increasingly important since the general sequence of auditory components is followed in the gross and environmental sound exercises. When lessons progress to the more difficult tasks in which speech sounds are employed, the listener has already developed some skill upon which to build.

The length of time involved in any given training period should be within the student's capability. The length of time should be gradually extended. Success, or approximations of success, should be appropriately rewarded. The reward must constitute something of value to the learner or it will not truly be reinforcing. If primary rewards such as edibles, tokens, or objects are used, they should be paired with pats, smiles, verbal approval, and similar social rewards which should replace the primary reward as quickly as the listener learns to value the social reward.

New tasks should be introduced in easy stages. Review of past landmarks should be a part of each session. Each session should terminate in success for the learner. When the learner displays difficulty with a given task, the teacher should move back to an exercise which can be handled successfully; then the new task should be broken down into the smallest possible increments. In such cases, it would be desirable to shorten the length of any given training session and provide more frequent presentations.

The response checklists incorporated into each step or lesson should be utilized faithfully. This is a specific way of ascertaining whether or not the learner has mastered the task being taught and is ready to progress to the next step. These checklists also serve as progress records. Use of both a checkmark and a date to indicate progress in terms of time invested will prove valuable.

Selected sample lessons are provided. They are intended to serve as a stimulus to the user of these materials. Many interesting lessons can easily be devised for any given step simply by varying the materials in terms of size, shape, color, texture, loudness, inflection, rhythm, etc. Other lesson variations may include role reversal, exploring new reward systems, and relating the lessons to practical everyday living activities. Learning to listen in specific ways will add interesting, new dimensions to the learner's life. He must be assisted to realize this. His efforts must be recognized and reinforced.

From gross sound exercises, these lessons progress to the use of live animal sounds. Just as gross sounds serve important purposes in these exercises, animal sounds provide a transitional step to vowel sounds. After teaching the listener animal sounds by using recordings of the actual animal production, they may then be presented with the human vocal mechanism. It is impossible to make animal sounds without employing vowels which are really speech sounds. Yet they are presented in a different context, and the learner is again assisted toward handling auditory speech input on a nonthreatening basis.

Following animal sounds; speech vowels, followed by syllables; words; phrases; sentences; and connected speech are presented. These increments involve the various components of auditory perception as they are known at the present time. Again, attention is drawn to the fact that this approximates the development of human language. The infant progresses from listening to environmental sounds to more differentiated listening and crying followed by babbling (syllables), lalling, echolalia, words, and finally to connected speech.

The exercises in this book have been used with varying degrees of success with both children and adults who have had normal, or nearly normal, hearing sensitivity but who have various suprathreshold problems. The aphasic, the language-disabled, the child of a minority culture, the emotionally disabled, the slow learner, and the neurologically handicapped have responded favorably to a concerted, consistent program based on these exercises. Parents have found them easy to understand and helpful in working with and managing children who often had been considered simply obstreperous when, in fact, they may have heard but failed to process adequately what was heard.

Speech and hearing therapists report these auditory perceptual training exercises to be helpful in working with the auditorially disabled and with articulation problems during the long, often frustrating, period of ear-training. Those who work with emotionally disturbed persons find these exercises to be useful in assisting the individual to function more comfortably in the sound environment from which he may have withdrawn.

With current emphasis on language disorders and the strong demands upon the university to provide pertinent, practical teacher training programs, this book could be a useful text for course work. It is recommended that opportunity to apply these materials in a practicum situation be a major part of such a course.

Persons who have been fitted with hearing aids should find these exercises helpful in adjusting to their new sound environment. It would be a considerable service were hearing aid representatives to make such a book available to their clients or, preferably, to provide a series of training classes under qualified guidance. This kind of structured assistance to new hearing aid users cannot be evaluated because it has never been studied in depth.

Teachers of hearing impaired children will find the sequence of auditory training procedures in this book to be appropriate for their students. It is logical to assume that in many cases, suprathreshold problems in addition to hearing loss, makes the learning process more difficult.

Other applications than those suggested will be identified as various disciplines examine and use these materials. Lessons should be modified to meet the specific needs of the learner. Each lesson should be interesting, practical, and presented in simple, clear language.

When the student falters on a given task, the teacher should be alert to the probability that she is approaching the crux of the problem in processing auditory imput. It must be re-emphasized that when this occurs, these specific tasks should not be discarded or bypassed but should be broken down into smaller, simpler steps which the listener can handle successfully. Gradually, then, the successes should be built upon until the desired response is obtained. Challenge ought, of course, to be a part of each lesson. However, each lesson should be terminated on a successful note.

Do not hurry the learner through the auditory perceptual tasks in this book. Do not assume that a single successful response indicates that a given task has been learned. Inconsistency is a common characteristic among individuals with auditory perceptual problems. Overlearning is, in most cases, preferable to incomplete learning. Review often. Vary the activities. Use the checklists. Make listening pleasant and rewarding. Both the teacher and the listener will begin to enjoy new dimensions in the sound environment.

The teacher should read through the Scope and Sequence Chart (Table 1) in order to gain some "feel" for the overall auditory perceptual training process. It will be noted that the materials needed for these lessons, are practical, simple, and inexpensive.

TABLE 1

AUDITORY PERCEPTUAL TRAINING PROGRAM
SCOPE AND SEQUENCE CHART

Level	*Type of Listening*	*Auditory Skills Involved*	*Materials*
I	Gross	Awareness, Sensation, Attention, Reception, Perception, (loudness, duration, pitch, quality, auditory memory, discrimination, sequencing, projection, localization, rhythm, separation.)	Drum, bell, rhythm instruments, crickets, any sound-producing object commonly found in the listener's environment. Tape recorder or other sound instruments such as radio, television, and record player.
II	Animal Sounds: a *Transitional Step* to Speech Vowel Sounds	All of the above to which has been added responsibility for attending to vocalized sound.	Taped recordings of live animal sounds for animals suggested below. Miniatures and pictures for common domesticated animals and birds. Sheep-duck-crow-pig-bird-mouse-horse-chicken-cat-dog-cow. Recorder, radio, T.V.

TABLE 1 (con't.)

Level	*Type of Listening*	*Auditory Skills Involved*	*Materials*
III	Listening for Vowels and Diphthongs	All of the above to which has been added responsibility for attending to vocalized sound in a speech context. Processing, Recall, Re-auditorization.	A series of pictures of lip configurations representing various vowel and diphthong sounds. Cards on which have been placed arrows to indicate upward or downward inflection. Rhythm cards.
IV	Listening for Speech Syllables	All of the above to which have been added consonant sounds, auditory blending, processing, recall, re-auditorization.	All of above for review. Cards with syllables imprinted in large, black manuscript form.
V	Discrimination for Spoken Words	All of the above. Auditory Closure.	All of above for review. Miniature objects and pictures of objects based on suggested vocabulary list.
VI	Discrimination for Phrases and Sentences	All of the above.	All of the above for review. Pictures to illustrate phrases and sentences.
VII	Discrimination for Connected Speech	All of the above.	All of the above.
VIII	Discrimination for Unstructured Auditory Materials	All of the above.	All of the above.

CHAPTER II

THE PROBLEM

THE FIRST PROBLEM arises in attempting to define auditory perceptual training. Traditionally, auditory training has implied a degree of hearing loss for which amplification was provided. Remediation, or auditory training, provided practice in listening and adjusting to the altered sound environment under amplification. Until recent years, little thought has been given to the logical, sequential order in which listening skills develop. Little attention had been given to the components involved in auditory perception and processing. Disabilities related to these factors may present severe problems in understanding, processing, and reproducing language either in the presence or absence of losses in hearing sensitivity. Jean Utley, in defining Auditory Training, states:

> The child who hears normally, is able to catch the meaning of sounds and to associate them with his other senses. He uses his hearing together with vision, feelings, tasting, smelling, in developing understanding, speech and language. The child whose hearing is impaired has to learn through the other senses and then be taught to associate them with his sense of hearing. We call this process Auditory Training.[1]

O'Neill, in discussing aural rehabilitation, writes, "Auditory training implies training with amplified sound."[2]

While such definitions and approaches to auditory training have created interest and pointed up unmet needs in the field of

[1] Utley, Jean: *What's Its Name.* Urbana, Ill., University of Illinois Press, 1950, p. 6.

[2] O'Neill, John J.: Aural Rehabilitation. In: *The Hard of Hearing.* Englewood Cliffs, New Jersey, Prentice-Hall, Inc., 1968.

auditory disorders, a more specific definition is required in a discussion of auditory perception and auditory perceptual disorders. Definitions which restrict auditory training exclusively to amplification for the hearing impaired may have an impeding effect on development of tests and remediation to meet the needs of individuals with auditory disorders of a supra-threshold nature. An operational definition of auditory perceptual training which allows for these kinds of problems seems appropriate.

> In the broadest sense, auditory perceptual training consists of a logical sequence of tasks involving listening, discrimination, adequate processing and reproduction of sound.[3]

Berry's definition of auditory perception seems comprehensive:

> Auditory perception of speech per se deals mainly with the temporal management of information from the input. It is a process by which one explains how a child's nervous system learns to comprehend and make use of auditory information.[4]

Mykelbust states that the many forms of auditory problems prevent many children from profiting academically.

> From the results of investigations of children with learning disabilities, it is apparent that auditory processes play a significant role in all verbal functioning, perhaps a leading role.[5]

As long ago as 1958, Hayes Newby suggested that auditory problems, other than hearing loss, would eventually require specific remediation.

> Some children seem to be deficient in . . . comprehending auditory verbal stimuli, even though their hearing acuity (sensitivity) is normal. In the future it may be necessary to establish listening classes for such children.[6]

[3] Heasley, Bernice E.: *A Programmed Manual of Auditory Training Exercises.* (Louisville, Ohio, The Stark County Department of Education Press, 1968, p. iii.

[4] Berry, Mildren Freburg: *Language Disorders of Children.* New York; Appleton-Century-Crofts, 1969, p. 59.

[5] Mykelbust, Helmer, R.: *Development and Disorders of Written Language,* New York, Grune & Stratton, 1965, Vol. I.

[6] Newby, Hayes, R.: *Audiology.* New York, Appleton-Century-Crofts 1964, p. 252.

Effective auditory functioning is dependent upon many factors, not necessarily related to hearing sensitivity. It is incumbent upon those persons engaged in the field of speech, hearing and language therapy to study and identify as many of these factors as possible. Remediation may be based upon observed behavior. There are few standardized tests to identify the problems which individuals may experience at supra-threshold levels. F. X. Blair has stated:

> Increased concern for children with special learning disabilities has helped to foster this philosophy of identifying the specific areas of the disability—Auditory, Visual, Tactile, Sensory, Perceptual, or Conceptual—which require remediation in order to permit the learner to realize his achievement potential.[7]

Descriptions of auditory behavior may result in identification of a variety of auditory disorders including reduced sensitivity to the sound spectrum. Other disorders which Blair suggests as target behaviors for remediation are:

> . . . phonemic discrimination difficulties, disruptions of the temporal sequencing of speech messages, and imperfect comprehension of spoken language.[8]

These auditory disruptions and their attendant learning disabilities have implications for the individual's life functioning. It was earlier stated that auditory processes may play a leading role in all verbal functioning. Few educators would contest this statement. Ruth Strickland, Reading Consultant, states it succinctly:

> The four ways in which language functions in school and in life are in listening, speaking, writing, and reading. Listening is the first to operate in the life of a normal individual and the one he uses more than any other. Yet emphasis on helping to listen is of comparatively recent emphasis. It stems from two facts—one is the realization that hearing and listening are not the same thing and that listening must be learned.[9]

[7] Blair, Francis X.: *Programming for auditorially disabled children. Except Child,* December, 1969, p. 260.

[8] *Ibid.*, p. 259.

[9] Strickland, Ruth G.: Learning to Listen. In: *The Language Arts In The Elementary School.* Boston, D. C. Heath & Company, 1957, p. 116.

Perhaps the dearth of remediation materials in the area of listening partially explains the numerous cases of correlated language problems in speech, reading, spelling, and writing, which have persisted in individuals who may or may not have hearing losses.

"Appropriate remediation," says John McLeod, in discussing reading expectancy, "can be indicated if relevant skills which are basic to, rather than merely correlated with, reading ability, are known. Current research suggests that such relevant basic skills are likely to be in terms of the ITPA model at the Automatic-Sequential level of organization and in the Auditory-Vocal Modality; e.g., phonemic discrimination, sound blending, immediate auditory memory span, etc."[10]

Educators in various fields related to language recognize this crucial nature of listening. Furthermore, listening is conceded to be a skill which must be taught. However, except in a general way, little remediation is available for disabled listeners. The process of listening is treated by the majority of educators either as a gestalt or is identified in terms of levels of listening. Only recently have educators—predominantly in the fields of Speech and Hearing Therapy, Audiology, and Language Therapy—attempted to identify the processes involved in sound perception, processing, and reproduction.

Hearing, one of our two distance senses, represents the major channel for learning. It is the first sense to develop in the newborn child. There are well-controlled studies to indicate that babies respond to sound even before birth.[11] Rough discrimination to sound pitch has been observed in the newborn at between one to four days following birth.[12] The child becomes aware of sound, he processes it, and, in some manner, stores it for future use. The exact manner in which this occurs is still largely a matter of speculation. We can provide explanatory constructs on paper; however, the actual process resists inspection. It is easier to

[10] McLeod, John: Reading expectancy from disabled learners. *Learn Disabil, 1*(2):104, 1968.

[11] McCandless, Boyd R.: *Children Behavior and Development.* New York, Holt, Rinehart, and Winston, Inc., 1967, p. 32

[12] *Ibid.*

observe the behavioral aspects of hearing than to explain the physiological events which culminate in the behavior.

Hearing has two separate, but related, aspects: sensitivity and perception. A loss of hearing sensitivity may be complicated by perceptual problems. However, an auditory perceptual problem may occur independently of reduced sensitivity. Normally, hearing sensitivity and perception function in a synchronized manner to preserve the well being of the individual and to result in language acquisition.

Limitations

This book is concerned with auditory perception as it is related to the acquisition and expression of verbal language. Discussion is limited to perceptual problems of a supra-threshold nature. While the book addresses itself to the normally hearing individual who suffers auditory perceptual problems, it is considered appropriate for the hearing impaired as well. Hearing losses seldom occur independently of other complicating factors.

Remediation Based Upon Behavior

The auditory mechanism is well protected within the skull. It defies ready inspection. Educators who are concerned with auditory perceptual disorders must, at this time, approach remediation of problems from a behavioral point of view. Sanders exemplifies such an approach:

> It is quite clear that sensory perception constitutes the basis of all forms of adaptive behavior.[13]

In planning remediation, one must consider not only the observed behavioral manifestations of auditory perception but also the natural developmental heirarchy of listening skills and language as they emerge in the young child.

> Lessons must be designed to progress from the discrimination of gross everyday environment sounds to the difficult task of discrimination of conversational speech under adverse listening conditions.[14]

[13] Sanders, Derek: *Aural Rehabilitation*. Englewood Cliffs, N.J., Prentice-Hall, Inc., 1971, p. 83.

[14] *Ibid.*, p. 87.

It may be assumed with a degree of confidence that auditory perception involves numerous distinct, but related, components.

> You see people, not rays of light, hear voices instead of the component sound vibrations. Your reaction is to *patterns* of stimuli; you are not usually aware of the component parts. Each of the pieces of this perceptual jigsaw may be looked at in isolation, but when you put them together they constitute a picture that you are only then able to recognize.[15]

There is growing interest in identification of the components of auditory perception. During routine hearing testing audiologists and speech clinicians may note patterns of confusion, abnormal rates of response, or abnormal patterns of consistency where no real impairment of sensitivity exists. Teachers or therapists may note, empirically, problems related to understanding of verbal language. Repeated observations may lead to identification of a disability related to a specific component of auditory perceptual functioning.

Certain pioneered tests of auditory discrimination have prompted interest in identifying components related to auditory perception. Well-known tests include *Wepman's Auditory Discrimination Test* which presents the listener with forty pairs of words, most of which are similar in sound, and a few of which are identical. The listener indicates whether the words are the same or different.[16]

The Boston University Speech Sound Discrimination Picture Test is a visual-auditory test. It consists of thirty-six cards, each of which has three pictures—two of which are similar or identical in sound. The listener responds by pointing to the pair of appropriate pictures which represent what the examiner verbalized.[17]

Mildred Templin has developed a test using pairs of nonsense syllables. The child responds by saying whether the sounds were the same or different.[18]

[15] *Ibid.*, p. 85.

[16] Wepman, J. M.: *Auditory Discrimination Test.* Chicago, 1958.

[17] *The Boston University Speech Sound Discrimination Picture Test.* Boston, 1955.

[18] Templin, Mildred C.: Study of sound discrimination ability of *elementary school pupils. J Speech Disord,* 8(2):132, 1943.

The Illinois Test of Psycholinguistic Abilities (ITPA) is of more recent origin and holds some promise for identifying areas which require remedial measures. A book of remediation materials based on this test has recently been published.[19]

The Goldman-Fristoe-Woodcock *Test of Auditory Discrimination,* also of recent origin, tests the ability of an individual to discriminate words in both the absence and presence of varying degrees of noise. This test further identifies the types of articulated phoneme errors.[20]

Carhart points out the desirability of constructing new tests of auditory functioning. He believes these tests would be more valid if they were constructed to simulate normal listening situations.

> The present need, if we are to assess practical efficiency in speech discrimination relatively directly, is for new tests which pit their test items against backgrounds that simulate the competition encountered in everyday situations.[21]

The Stark County Department of Education, Stark County, Ohio, conducts a hearing conservation program in which the hearing of approximately ten thousand elementary-age school children is screened each year. This is accomplished by a mobile hearing laboratory which is equipped to screen the hearing of four children simultaneously. The Zenith Visual Auditory Screen for Children (VASC), installed in serial arrangement, has been the testing instrument. Children failing the initial hearing screen are immediately provided pure-tone retests in a two-room, sound-treated suite on the mobile unit.

The large numbers of children involved in this hearing conservation program have identified differences in auditory functioning among the children. Significant patterns of behavior, especially among younger children, were observed by the Coordinating Audiologist during the five years of the program's operation.[22]

[19] Bush, Wilma Jo and Giles, Marian Taylor: *Aids to Psycholinguistic Teaching.* Columbus, Ohio, Charles S. Merrill Publishing Co., 1969.

[20] Goldman, Ronald, Fristoe, Macalyne, and Woodcock, Richard W.: *Test of Auditory Discrimination.* Minnesota, American Guidance Service, 1970.

[21] Carhart, Raymond: *Problems in the measurement of speech discrimination. Arch Otolaryngol,* 82:260, 1965.

[22] Dickerhoof, Richard G., Coordinating Audiologist

A small, but consistent, percentage of children who failed the VASC screening test, particularly at lower levels of intensity, were found upon pure-tone retest to have normal hearing sensitivity. However, consultation with classroom teachers revealed that many of these children have concommitant problems with reading, spelling, writing, and understanding directions.

In cooperation with the VASC manufacturer, The Director of Audiological Services,[23] The Stark County Supervisor of Speech and Hearing Therapy,[24] and The Coordinating Audiologist constructed a test to measure the effects of competing signals at varying intensities upon a primary message among young elementary age school children. This Test of Auditory Separation Ability (TASA) is presently being administered to a number of first-through fourth grade children in the Stark County Schools in order to standardize the levels at which competing signals constitute learning blocks.

Individuals with auditory perceptual problems often display symptoms which appear similar to those of individuals with losses of hearing sensitivity; they may not respond to acoustic stimuli at normal levels of intensity. They may display difficulty in locating the sound source. Hyperactivity and short attention span are shared factors. Poor auditory memory and memory span and poor sequencing ability are also factors in common. It may be necessary to repeat directions more frequently in order to assure the listener's comprehension. Speech sounds may be reversed. Letters in spelling and writing may be reversed. Educational achievement may not be commensurate with measured potential. In fact, measured potentials (I.Q.) may be invalid.

Earlier it was stated that the auditory channel has proved difficult to study. Results of hearing tests do not really provide adequate information about the channel of hearing. These tests chart the respondent's motor response to the acoustic stimuli which were presented. Audiograms may or may not reflect accurate representations of the sound stimuli which was presented or which the individual received. It is, however, less difficult to

[23] Briskey, Robert

[24] Briskey, Robert, Heasley, Bernice E., and Dickerhoof, Richard G.

test for hearing sensitivity than to test for auditory perception. The need for refined standardized tests of auditory perceptual functioning and for auditory perceptual remediation has been clearly advanced. It may be impractical to wait for conclusive tests to verify the presence of auditory perceptual problems which are behaviorally apparent. Auditorially disabled individuals are in need of help now. Remedial materials for auditory perceptual problems of a supra-threshold nature may, in fact, be of considerable value in the construction of identification measures.

The remedial materials in this book have been field tested but have not been subjected to controlled clinical testing. This outline of auditory perceptual remediation is presented as one approach.

In all probability, very few of the components involved in auditory perception, processing, and reproduction are known at the present time. This must not deter educators from developing remediation techniques for problems which are clearly identifiable in terms of behavior.

CHAPTER III

COMPONENTS OF AUDITORY PERCEPTION

In undertaking the task of identifying and defining certain of the known components of auditory perception, every attempt has been made to arrange them in a heirarchy which follows the normal developmental sequence of skill acquisition in the child. The following taxonomy is suggested.

1. Awareness of sound
2. Auditory attention
3. Auditory attention span
4. Localization of sound
5. Discrimination for sound
6. Auditory memory
7. Auditory memory span
8. Sound sequencing ability
9. Auditory projection ability
10. Auditory separation
11. Auditory blending
12. Auditory closure
13. Re-auditorization

Generally, the above suggested order will be observed as the remediation exercises move from gross sound to speech stimuli. It was noted earlier that the above components may represent only a fraction of those which may play either discrete or interacting roles in the sound perception-processing-reproduction phenomena leading to language acquisition. For purposes of this book, only those components which can be behaviorally observed and described are given attention.

However incomplete an outline of auditory perceptual factors may be, there is no dispute among educators regarding the importance of listening skills.

> Practice in listening and recognition and the acquisition of the rudiments of motor skill are both preparatory stages leading to the development of speech in its full sense, that is, to the learning of the language system.[1]

Awareness of Sound

Awareness may be defined as the ability to recognize and respond to the presence or absence of sound. As in all components of perception, we shall accept as evidence of success the respondent's ability to correctly discriminate and identify the stimuli. Sanders states:

> Before a person in a communication situation is ready to receive a speech signal, he must be motivated to do so. The motivation to listen is important, since it gives rise to auditory-perceptual expectancy.[2]

Awareness of the signal must be ascertained even before the motivation to listen may be expected of the respondent. Blair points out the basic need of an individual to be sensitized to the raw sensory data of his environment.

> Fundamental needs of survival and adaptability as well as prelinguistic and precognitive stages of development are served. Basic environment contact is made.[3]

However, some children with apparently normal hearing acuity, for a variety of reasons seem insensitive to environmental, non-speech sounds or signals. These presymbolic stages of audition must be developed to a meaningful degree before the more subtle speech and language sounds can be processed. These are highly essential stages in normal human development.[4]

[1] Fry, D. B.: The development of the phonological system in the normal and the deaf child. In: *The Genesis of Language*. Cambridge, Mass., The M.I.T. Press, 1968, p. 193.

[2] Sanders, Derek: *Aural Rehabilitation*. Englewood Cliffs, New Jersey, Prentice-Hall, Inc., 1971 p. 96.

[3] Blair, Francis X.: *Programming for auditorially disabled children. Except Child*, December 1969, p. 259.

[4] *Ibid.*, p. 260.

Awareness of sound source must first be established with a high degree of consistency as the foundation for more involved listening. In working with the auditorially disabled person, the teacher or therapist should ascertain that this first basic step is well established before proceeding to subsequent exercises. Even though the individual may already indicate sound awareness by responding to the signal, awareness tasks can be utilized as a means of establishing a set of expected responses from the listener. These easy tasks have the added importance of providing him with some success upon which to build.

At the awareness level, the infant responds first to loudness and duration.[5] Remediation should begin with sufficiently loud and long signals to assure awareness. Both loudness and duration may be reduced as the listener gains skill as indicated by appropriate, consistent responses.

Auditory Attention

Attention may be linked with *intention* to lend oneself to the task at hand; listening. Blair, in delineating his heirarchy of auditory receptive behavior, identifies attention with a listening set under signal acceptance.[6]

Having received the signal, the listener accepts responsibility for further processing of the stimulus by increased attention. Auditory attention is necessary to sound processing. It is an aspect of auditory perception which would seem to improve as a result of programmed listening exercises combined with Behavior Modification (Operant Conditioning) techniques.

The important difference between awareness (hearing) and Auditory Attention is well described by Blair:

> The level of *perceptual organization* involves in the first instance a prerequisite set which we are calling attention readiness. This function distinguishes hearing from listening and assumes on the part of the organism a predisposition to essential auditory behavior . . . But as we have come to realize, the organism must of necessity "tune in" to relevant aspects of the environmental information avail-

[5] McCandless, Boyd R.: *Children Behavior and Development.* New York, Holt, Rinehart & Winston, Inc. 1967, p. 32.

[6] Blair, Francis X.: *Op. Cit.*, p. 259.

able, particularly those related to social relationships. It is assumed that early in life the language example of significant adults surrounding the child becomes highly relevant and the child learns to selectively attend to those messages, which initially probably only communicate an ill-defined state of well-being. Gradually, associative meaning to the world of object referents is established and symbolization begins its development.[7]

Auditory Attention Span

Simply defined, Auditory Attention Span will be referred to as the individual's ability to attend selectively for increased lengths of time to a task or series of tasks. It is obvious that auditory attention span, auditory memory, and auditory memory span are inter-related acoustic functions. Tasks intended to lead to improved skills in one area would, almost inevitably, lead to improved concommitant skills in related areas.

> Memory may become weakened for immediate situations because of a primary defect of attention.[8]

Maintenance of records in the Auditory Perceptual Exercises, will show evidence of increased ability to attend over a reasonable period of time. For some individuals, the progress may be apparent within days. Others may require several weeks of work before appreciable attention span is manifest. Improvement of attention span may be related to the work setting. If the lessons are highly structured, and if distracting stimuli are screened out, at least in the initial stages, improved attention span may be quickly apparent.

Localization of Sound

Localization involves the ability to identify the direction from which a sound or series of sounds originated. The importance of this sound component may be inferred from the early age at which this skill develops.

[7] Blair, Francis X.: Language Disorders; A Dimension of Learning Disabilities. Seminars in Psychiatry, August, 1969.

[8] Berry, Mildred F. and Eisonson, Jon: *Speech Disorders.* New York, Appleton-Century-Crofts, Inc., 1956, p. 395.

> The child relates hearing and vision between two and three months of age: when he hears a sound he attempts to locate the source visually by turning his head to see where the sound is coming from.[9]

The problems of localization failure in relation to language development or even to language usage are more important than would first appear to be the case. The individual who cannot normally localize the sound source, stands to lose a considerable portion of the signal, or verbal message, during the time he has spent on this attempt.

Localization of sound for the hearing-aid user requires that the signal be received at both sides of the head. A single hearing aid, fitted with a Y-Cord, would render the individual incapable of participating in this task since all sound is received through a common microphone and, therefore, from a single direction.

Discrimination For Sound

An operational, if simplistic, definition of discrimination may be described as the ability to recognize and respond appropriately to similarities and differences in sound. Probably the first form of sound discrimination would be in the area of pitch. M. M. Lewis notes that:

> 1. At an early stage (before the infant is about nine months old), the child shows discrimination, in a broad way, among different patterns of expression in intonation.
> 2. When the total pattern . . . the phonetic form together with intonational form . . . is made effective by training, at first the intonational rather than the phonetic form dominates the child's responses.[10]

This seems a logical criterion for spending the necessary amount of time on obtaining consistent responses to structured lessons based on gross or environmental sound stimuli. Lewis elaborates further:

> 3. Then the phonetic pattern becomes the dominant feature in evoking the specific response; but while the function of the intona-

[9] Mykelbust, Helmer R.: *Auditory Disorders in Children*. New York, Grune & Stratton, 1954, p. 90.

[10] Lewis, M. M.: *Infant Speech*, New York, Humanities Press, 1951, pp. 115–116.

tional pattern may be considerably subordinated, it certainly does not vanish.[11]

The dimensions of sound include frequency (pitch), intensity (loudness), duration (rate), and phase (quality). Discrimination tasks, then, must include these four dimensions whether the stimuli be gross sound or speech sound.

Sanders, in discussing testing of auditory discrimination, suggests the following heirarchy:

Testing vowel-sound discrimination.
Testing Consonant sound discrimination.
Testing Multiple Choice Word Discrimination.
Testing Auditory Discrimination Under Conditions of Noise.

The same factors involved in the learning of gross sounds discrimination are valid in the learning of speech perception.[12]

The above heirarchy for testing of speech sound discrimination does not take into account the many steps involved before the individual arrives at the point where he can even provide test results. It is necessary to develop discrimination, beginning with gross sound stimuli and progressing gradually to the more difficult sounds—speech.

Auditory Memory

Auditory memory is the ability to remember the characteristics of a given sound or series of sounds. Auditory memory is involved with virtually every task associated with perception, processing, and reproduction of sound. Several of the dimensions of auditory memory are treated separately because, behaviorally, they may be observed and described as distinct entities of the whole. For example, auditory memory span, sequencing ability, projection, separation, blending, and closure are factors closely related to and dependent upon memory. These factors will be discussed in a later portion of this chapter.

The individual whose short-term memory, or memory for immediate recall, is abnormally short will experience severe learning difficulties. Sound may eventually become so lacking in mean-

11 *Ibid.*
12 Sanders, *op. cit.*, p. 107.

ing that he may tune it out altogether in time. At best, it will take a much longer time for the individual with this type of impairment to process sound. The therapist or teacher may find it necessary to spend considerable time on auditory memory inasmuch as further progress is dependent upon the acquisition of this skill among auditorially disabled individuals.

> Performance operates under constraints of memory, which is finite, and time, which must be kept up with.[13]

Auditory Memory Span

Auditory Memory Span refers to the individual's ability to remember for increasing lengths of time the characteristics of a given sound or series of sounds. It is probably closely associated with auditory imagery, a concept which has been given little attention. Implications for further research on auditory imagery, auditory recall, and re-authorization suggest themselves.

Auditory Memory Span and Auditory Attention Span probably complement each other in the heirarchy of developing auditory perceptual skills. There is ample evidence that auditory sequencing ability also plays a significant role in Auditory Memory Span. Again referring to Blair:

> The comprehension process in such an instance would seem to involve an auditory "holding action" pending completion of the statement. This is frequently verified when certain of these children attempt to carry out the commands individually *as they are given* as if finding it impossible to delay the response until the directions are completed by the examiner.[14]

Tasks intended to help the individual improve memory and memory span ought to begin at basic receptive levels:

> Sanders demonstrates that children with primary expressive language disorders have poor memory span for simple nouns and the deficiency prevails whether the response required of the subjects is verbal or a simple motor response to pictures of the units presented. The indication from this study is that success with the memory span

[13] McNeil, David: Development Psycholinguistics. Smith, Frank and Miller, George A., (Eds.): *The Genesis of Language*. Cambridge, M.I.T. Press, 1900, 1966, p. 17.

[14] Blair, *op. cit.*

task is more related to input or receptive language integrity than to output or response.[15]

Teaching such a task as auditory memory span with gross sound instruments may reduce the possibility of echolalic responses which might be precipitated in verbal tasks at the later word level where the listener is requested to repeat a series of words or digits.

Auditory Sequencing Ability

The ability to identify a series of sounds in correct, respective order is called sound sequencing. This is an over-simplification of a complex task which involves several auditory perceptual dimensions and which is critical in the ultimate development of verbal language.

The significance of serial order (temporal sequencing) of input stimuli is clarified by Hirsch:

> The patterns that one distinguishes and recognizes in hearing are formed or articulated in time, and these temporal patterns are rather peculiar to hearing. Furthermore, language, as received by the ear and not by the eye, is similarly formed in time. Not only can we note that speech consists of elements and element combinations that are themselves temporal patterns, but also the structure of language involves, to an enormous extent, storage, perceptual stretching, and relation-making over rather long extents of time.[16]

Monsees, in reporting on disabilities of Aphasics (persons who suffer language disorders), states:

> Research showing a definite relationship between temporal sequence perception and aphasia in adults reported by Efron (1963) was replicated with aphasic children by Lowe and Campbell (1965) with similar findings.[17]

In the experience of the author, Auditory Sequencing Ability along with problems of Auditory Attention and Attention Span,

[15] *Ibid.*, p. 11.

[16] Hirsch, Ira J.: Information Processing in imput channels for speech and language; The significance of serial order of stimuli. In Millikan, C. H. & Darley, F. L. (Eds.): *Brain Mechanisms Underlying Speech and Language.* New York, Grune & Stratton, 1967, p. 21.

[17] Monsees, Edna K.: Temporal sequence and expressive language disorders. *Except Child,* October, 1968; p. 142.

and Auditory Memory and Auditory Memory Span, rank high as factors common to the auditorially disabled individual. Monsees again provides information on research in this area:

> About thirty years ago, Orton (1937) published his findings on children with various types of language disorders and concluded that the one factor that seemed to be common to all of them was "a difficulty in repicturing or rebuilding in the order of presentation, sequences of letters, of sounds, or of units of movement.
>
> Specifically with reference to what he termed "developmental motor aphasia," Orton said that the major difficulty in these cases was a result almost without exception of an inability to blend sounds which the subject could reproduce in isolation.
>
> McGinnis (1963) also reported that "motor aphasic children" have difficulty in memory for sequence of sounds that they are able to produce in isolation.
>
> There has been no reported research in the professional literature of audiology and speech pathology, to the author's knowledge, to support the clinical observations of Orton (1937) and McGinnis (1963), nor have there been studies of the relationship of poor intelligibility of spoken language and temporal sequencing difficulties.[18]

Auditory Sequencing, then, is a critical factor in the processing of auditory perceptual input. Intact sequencing ability leads to language development and verbal skill. Conversely, a disability in Sequencing will delay or prevent language acquisition and expression.

> The reception of spoken language signals involves a sequential series of acoustic events occurring along a time dimension. Evidence gathered from diagnostic work and the teaching of aphasic children indicates that the integrity of this function may be critical to the proper comprehension of spoken language.[19]

Disorders may be related to nonverbal sound reception of the individual. The implications are that, prior to requiring ordering of speech sounds, the auditorially perceptually impaired individual should be provided the necessary practice in ordering nonspeech sounds.

[18] *Ibid.*
[19] *Ibid.*

> Stated in another way, the associative level of comprehension may be deleteriously affected by pre-symbolic factors relating to imput to the auditory system.[20]

Sequencing, along with other auditory perceptual skills is probably present in varying degrees among the impaired individual.

> A child having a severe auditory-vocal sequencing input disability may understand much of his everyday language if he is not overloaded, i.e., if verbal messages are provided in small units of information "chunks." Children of this type cannot track along sentences but must be given sentences of three to four words, for example.[21]

Sequencing skills often appear to resist improvement. This is not surprising when one considers the dimensions of auditory perceptual tasks involved in sequencing ability: Awareness, Attention, Localization, Discrimination, Memory, Rhythm, and perhaps also Separation, Projection, Blending, Closure, and re-auditorization. Improvement may be observed after a time, however. This improvement will be recorded in the progress record which should be a part of each lesson.

Auditory Projection

Projection, as it relates to auditory perception, must be distinguished from the traditional psychological and psychiatric meaning ascribed to this word.

> There are a wide variety of meanings given to the term *projection* by different psychiatrists and psychologists, but one given by Norman Cameron probably encompasses some of the main ideas that most of us have when we use the term. "By projection we mean ascribing our own attributes to other persons, groups, objects and symbols . . ." [22]

In the case of auditory projection, our connotation and denotation is concerned with normal, rather than with abnormal phenomena. Projection, for our purposes, will be defined as the ability of the individual to attend to and process sound signals which

[20] *Ibid.*, p. 8.
[21] *Ibid.*, pp. 8–9.
[22] Washburne, Chandler: Projection and role-taking. In: Lennon, E. James (Ed.): *Acta Symbolica.* Akron, Ohio, University of Akron, Fall 1971, p. 2.

originate from increasingly greater distances from the listener. Projection is of vital importance to the individual's survival and ultimately to his social well-being, since it normally leads to the ability to "scan" the auditory environment. Scanning for danger signals as well as scanning for socially reinforcing signals is a common auditory activity.

The importance of this ability to project one's listening (or to stretch one's ability to listen) is seen readily in the auditorially disabled child who is able to attend when he is seated in close proximity to the sound signal, but who, upon being some distance away appears to "decay out."

Perhaps Auditory Projection Ability is related to Separation Ability which is subsequently discussed as another component of auditory perception.

> Our orientation in space is also dependent upon the integration of information from external and internal sensory mechanism. From these sources we obtain not only information relevant to posture and balance, but also information concerning the position of our body relative to objects around us. The role of hearing in spatial orientation is, perhaps, underestimated.[23]

Auditory Separation

Auditory Separation is related to foreground-background sound discrimination. It is defined here as the ability to attend to a primary sound signal in the presence of extraneous (competing) sound stimuli.

Sanders equates the importance of closure and figure-ground:

> We also note that we are influenced in what we perceive by our previous experience. How do we organize these multitudinous stimuli in order to make possible the designation of meaning? In communication two phenomena are particularly important in this process: figure-ground and closure.[24]

Perception of the figure (primary) stimuli from the ground (competing) stimuli is applicable to both the channels of vision and hearing.

[23] Sanders, *op. cit.*, p. 84.
[24] *Ibid.*, p. 85.

It (figure-ground perception) makes it possible for you to attend to a particular sound source against a background or other environmental noises and to shift your attention from one sound source to another.[25]

Auditory Separation is also closely allied with auditory attention, for attention implies a state in which the individual lends himself to the task of listening for and responding to a specific stimulus or stimuli to the exclusion of others. In order to maintain attention, he must inhibit potential interfering auditory stimuli. Word, context and social meaning influences this function to a great extent. For example, an individual normally separates and identifies his own name in the presence of interfering stimuli. This phenomenon is worthy of further research.

When one observes the functional interacting auditory perceptual factors, one is impressed with the magnitude of language acquisition. The important role of Auditory Separation permits the individual to respond selectively to a multitude of choices among auditory stimuli.

Auditory Blending

Roswell and Chall have developed a test for Auditory Blending ability. In discussing the purpose of the test, a definition may be inferred:

This test gives an estimate of a pupil's ability to blend sounds, auditorily into whole words whether or not he has learned to associate the sounds with the corresponding letters. Thus it is particularly useful for judging the ease or difficulty that pupils will experience in phonics instruction.[26]

Blending is the reverse process of syllabication.

Syllabication consists of the ability to divide words into syllables. Whereas *Auditory Blending* entails the facility to combine isolated syllables into words . . . It is not uncommon to see children with disturbances of written language that are related to inabilities of this type.[27]

[25] *Ibid.*, p. 87.

[26] Roswell, Florence G. and Chall, Jeanne S.: *Auditory Blending Test,* Manual of Instructions. New York, Essay Press, p. 1.

[27] Mykelbust, Helmer R.: *Development and Disorders of Written Language* (ch. II) p. 32. Grune & Stratton, N.Y. and London, 1965.

Auditory Closure

The ability to recognize and synthesize discrete parts of a sound production into a whole production is called Auditory Closure. For example: to reconstruct the parts (c-t) into the whole word (cat).

Auditory Closure has implications for language and speech reception and production.

At the word production level, Bannatyne's definition permits greater latitude of definition, and therefore presents a broader range to consider in providing remediation.

> Auditory Closure . . . is the ability to identify the true or accurate pronunciation of a word; which has been spoken in a slovenly way or even mis-pronounced. For example, if I say *uhni*verse, most of you will immediately realize I should have said universe, or if I say a*uto*matic, I should have said auto*mat*ic. In many reading disability cases, children seem to find it difficult to close on their own slightly erroneous pronunciation of specific words, and training to improve this may be undertaken by the staff speech therapist.[28]

Subvocalization

The facet of auditory perception cannot really be observed or counted. However, in discussing the value of subvocalizing sound with auditorially disabled individuals, subvocalization appears to be a mechanism or reinforcing auditory processing. There appear to be two facets to subvocalization:

1. Thinking about and attempting to "hold" the sound stimulus in mind. This may be related to auditory imagery and re-auditorization.
2. In addition to the above, to move the articulators without sound production to reinforce the heard vocal patterns.

Stendler points out that subvocalization may play an important role in language acquisition.

> Assuming that some degree of subvocal rehearsal (for vocal "imagining") is possible in small children, we can also explain why it is

[28] Bannatyne, Alex D.: Matching Remedial Methods With Specific Deficits. PROCEEDINGS, 1967 Internation Convocation on Children and Young Adults With Learning Disabilities, Home for Crippled Children, Pittsburgh, Pennsylvania, July, 1967, p. 156.

that children often "come out" as we say, with well-formed words which we have never before heard them attempt to utter.[29]

Reauditorization

The unvoiced recollection and "holding" of a sound production, whether at the gross sound level or at the speech level, is referred to in this context as reauditorization. Auditory memory is involved in this accomplishment. At the speech level, it may occur at several of the levels in the infant's heirarchy of speech development landmarks. Very early the infant may attempt to imitate an inflection pattern heard by a significant person in his environment. He is encouraged and rewarded for doing this when the adult imitates the infant's own production. This act of mutual reinforcement leads normally to language, word, and sentence acquisition. In order to accomplish this facet, the infant must remember and hold for reference and future reproduction, the acoustic characteristics of the signal. The Speech Clinician knows the value of the reauditorization process. One of the critical steps in speech correction is the long, tedious step of ear-training the speech-impaired individual to his own production as well as to the therapist's production. Through reauditorization of the model patterns, he learns to discriminate his own speech productions. The therapist will request him to remember his correct production and practice it in his thinking for a given period before she asks him to practice alone, aloud.

Reauditorization, as a remediation tool, should be built into all lessons which involve speech sounds. The auditorially disabled individual should be encouraged to remember and hold the production for the clinician or teacher. He should be encouraged to assume the "teacher role" in order to reinforce his production at the propitious time.

Reauditorization is probably a similar function of visual imagery. It was earlier suggested that reauditorization is probably closely associated with subvocalization.

It would seem that subvocalization, auditory imagery, and reauditorization may, in fact, be progressions of the same process.

[29] Martin, William E. and Stendler, Celia Burns: *Readings in Child Development.* New York, Harcourt, Brace and Company, 1954, p. 287.

The author has attempted in this chapter to identify, define, and discuss an heirarchy of auditory perceptual components. Now let us turn our attention to the remedial exercises which have been developed in an attempt to help the auditorially disabled individual improve his subnormal listening skills.

CHAPTER IV

GROSS AUDITORY PERCEPTUAL TRAINING EXERCISES

It was pointed out earlier that exercise in Gross Auditory Perceptual Training serve several important purposes:

1. These exercises establish a foundation upon which to develop more difficult tasks.
2. These exercises do not involve speech sounds, which to some individuals may be emotionally rejected. Therefore, they provide the learner a "set" which is success oriented.
3. These exercises establish a way of teaching with noncomplex materials.
4. They establish a way for the listener to respond.
5. These exercises establish the sequence of auditory perceptual components which will be given attention in the more difficult exercises which follow.

It would be erroneous to omit the gross auditory perceptual exercises. Depending upon the ease with which the learner progresses in these lessons, the teacher may progress fairly rapidly to the more complex, speech sounds. Should this strategy be followed, portions of gross exercises may then be employed on a review basis.

The teacher should present lessons which are simple and concrete until it is apparent that the child can function at a more complex level. Written comments following each lesson are highly valuable. In addition, a checklist to indicate whether or not success was achieved on any given lesson should be a part of each lesson plan. The checklist is based on the tasks which are required in the plan. When he is able to correctly perform three of any four given tasks, the next lesson should be presented. The portion of the lesson which was not entirely successful should be placed on a review basis until skill develops.

GROSS AUDITORY TRAINING EXERCISES

Step I. *Awareness of Gross Sound*

The majority of individuals will require only brief practice on this step. A few, however, who may have psychologically "tuned sound out," may require concerted work in order to respond to a gross sound signal.

A. Develop awareness of gross sound by seating the individual very close to a record player, tape recorder, television, or radio. Turn the volume up loudly enough that he can recognize when it is turned *on* or *off*. Place his hand on the instrument so he can get additional help from the channel of vibration. Turn it off and on several times until the listener consistently indicates awareness of the presence or absence of sound by a designated method of response.

B. Repeat the above exercise but request the individual to either raise his finger or drop a bead or bottle cap into a box when he hears the sound. It is permissible for him to watch this step. This is an important preconditioning task for helping the listener respond for the more difficult tasks and for pure tone hearing testing.

C. Obscure the listener's vision and repeat the exercise. Keep a written record of the number of trials and successful responses. This will help in evaluating progress.

D. Using music from the record player, or other source, at a sufficiently loud level, assist the individual to perform rhythmic body movement. Clapping, arm and leg, or whole body movement may be involved.

SAMPLE LESSON PLAN FOR AWARENESS OF GROSS SOUNDS

Objective: Consistent listener awareness of gross sound stimuli.

Materials: Radio
Box and several colored buttons.

Activity:
1. Demonstrate what is expected of the child by performing the following tasks:
   a. Turn the radio to the On position. Volume should be comfortably loud. Immediately, upon hearing the sound, drop a button into

the box which is placed on a table between the teacher and the listener.

b. After several demonstrations, assist the listener to drop a button into the box as soon as the sound is heard.

c. Reverse roles. Allow "listener" to manipulate the radio.

Teacher's Comments

Checklist:

______ 1. Observes and seems to understand what is expected after having task demonstrated several times.

______ 2. Is able, consistently, to demonstrate awareness of sound by dropping button into box each time radio is turned ON.

______ 3. Demonstrates understanding of process by assuming the teacher role successfully.

Step II. *Development of Auditory Attention Through Discrimination for Gross Sound*

A. Under comfortable loud amplification, present *two* sounds such as a drum and bell. Ask the individual to identify the source of sound. Do this by placing the instruments on a table which is comfortably low for the listener. Pick up the drum, and say, "This is a drum." Sound it. Allow the listener to sound it as he holds it near his ear. Now instruct him to replace it on the table and to leave it. Repeat the process for the bell. Demonstrate how the listener should respond by performing the task yourself. Put your own head down on the table, for a child; for an adult, simply close your eyes. Sound one of the instruments. Now, tap yourself on the head or arm as a signal that you may now "look." Rather quickly, choose the correct instrument which you sounded. *Do* take time, however, to look at both instruments. This is important in setting the pattern so the individual does not fall into the habit of guessing or making random response.

Repeat the process with the Listener doing the work. When he is looking at the instruments, be very careful not to glance at the instrument which you sounded. Hearing impaired individuals are very quick to pick up visual clues.

B. Develop the ability to localize sound by sounding the instruments in different parts of the room. The respondent, whose vision would be obscured while ONE instrument was sounded, may point to the direction from which the sound came, or point and also name the sound he heard.

C. When the child can discriminate consistently between the two instruments, increase the number to three and repeat the procedure.

D. Increase the number of instruments to four, then five, following the same procedure.

E. Vary the instruments, using any of five. We are presenting loud, unlike sounds at this point.

F. Repeat all above exercises and gradually reduce the volume.

G. Repeat all above exercises using prerecorded sounds which are fed through the tape recorder. Good use may be made of household and environmental sounds such as vacuum, horns, airplanes, etc.

For the Hearing Impaired

1. Repeat all exercises, using only the individual's hearing aid as a means of amplification.
2. Repeat all above exercises to the extent that it is possible without amplification.
3. Using amplification, repeat the above exercises against background noise which is gradually increased in loudness.

SAMPLE LESSON PLAN FOR DISCRIMINATION OF GROSS SOUND

Objectives: Correct listener identification of any of five unlike sound instruments under conditions of reduced volume.

Materials: Drum, bell, whistle, glass and spoon, band-aid box containing stones. (Band-aid box should be glued closed to prevent attempts to open the box and disrupt the lesson).

Activity:

1. The teacher will sound each of the five instruments and name them.
2. The teacher will hand each of the five instruments to the listener, request that he "sound" them, name them, and remember the sound.

3. The teacher will request the listener to turn his back to the instruments. She will sound one. (The teacher will have preconditioned the listener not to turn toward the instruments until tapped by the teacher).
4. The teacher will say "ready" indicating that the listener may turn and identify the instrument.
5. Express approval of correct response.
6. Sound each of the instruments in the same way. Be careful NOT to look at the instrument which was sounded.
7. Repeat above exercises with gradually reduced levels of loudness.
8. Reverse roles.

Teacher's
Comments

Checklist:

——— 1. Listener is able to identify anyone of five sound instruments correctly, four of five times.

——— 2. Listener is able to identify any one of five sound instruments correctly, four of five times, when the sound is very soft.

——— 3. Listener demonstrates understanding of the process by assuming the teacher role and providing the lesson correctly.

Step III. *Discrimination for Localization of Sound*

Any individual who has been in a situation where several persons are speaking or where there are a variety of sounds at fairly loud levels knows the problems involved in attempting to respond to an unexpected signal. Frequently, in his attempts to locate the sound source, the individual misses much, or all, of the message. Inasmuch as there is a dearth of information on this factor, there is little evidence that the powers of localization can be improved. On the other hand, there is no evidence that improvement of this skill, through a carefully constructed series of lessons, cannot be accomplished. Very often, simply being aware of the problem may make the individual more localization-conscious, thus improving performance.

Before undertaking a program to improve localization of sound ability, it would be determined by a qualified audiologist whether a unilateral hearing loss may be the cause of subnormal localization ability. An individual with such a hearing loss would be unable to improve his localization ability unless he is provided some means of cross amplification.

A. Station two or three persons in various locations in the room. Each should have identical sound instruments. One should sound the instrument. The listener's vision should be obscured. The listener should indicate from which direction the sound came.
B. Gradually decrease the volume and repeat the above exercises.
C. Repeat exercises, introducing a short time lapse.
D. Gradually increase the time lapse in order to develop memory for localization of sound.
E. Gradually move to a distance of two feet from the listener. Gradually increase the distance. This should be presented comfortably loudly. This will assist the listener to project listening for localized sound.

For the Hearing Impaired.

In order to develop this skill, the listener must be fitted with true binaural amplification, or he must function with none at all. A hearing aid or an auditory training unit with a Y-cord, or a unit served by a common microphone, will cancel out localization of sound.

Having fitted the listener with a true binaural hearing aid, or without amplification of any kind, help him to develop skill in locating the source of two identical instruments such as clickers. Begin with loud sounds very close to one ear or the other. Gradually move away from him until he can identify whether it is on one side or the other, at a short distance, on the table, or under the table.

Step IV. *Development of Auditory Memory Span*

Although the process of memory and auditory imagery is inherent in virtually all of these exercises, it is very important that the auditorially disabled person be given specific help and techniques to assist him in developing skills for remembering.

Auditory imagery is the ability to reconstruct and hold in mind the heard sound after the signal has ceased. Auditory memory and auditory imagery appear to be a part of the same process. They will not be treated differentially in this outline.

A. Secure four or five small tins in which have been placed such items as:
   1. Paper clips in one sealed tin
   2. Wooden pegs in a sealed tin
   3. Nuts and bolts
   4. pins
   5. bottle caps

   The teacher should begin with two of the described sound instruments. Sound one, allow a short time lapse, then request the listener to sound both and identify (from memory) which the teacher had sounded. After a practice lesson, the listener's vision should be obscured. The number of instruments and the length of time lapse should be increased as the listener demonstrates skill by consistent, appropriate responses.

B. Repeat the above exercises with gradually decreasing volume.

C. Repeat the above procedures with prerecorded sounds. Slight amplification, through the use of an auditory training unit, may help to create an increased awareness of sound. This should be abandoned when the listener demonstrates sufficient skill to function without it.

D. Gradually move a distance from the listener to force him to project his listening in terms of physical distance.

E. Repeat above exercises against background noise which is gradually increased in volume.

For the Hearing Impaired:

Present all exercises with the listener's hearing aid at a comfortably loud level. Gradually reduce the intensity to encourage him to project his listening.

SAMPLE LESSON PLAN FOR AUDITORY MEMORY SPAN

Objectives: 1. Improvement of memory for gross sound stimuli.
2. Increased memory span for similar gross sound instruments.

Materials: Two bells. These should be somewhat different in

pitch, but not as obviously different as a large brass bell and a small brass bell.

Activity: It is assumed that the listener has successfully identified one of among several instruments when he is requested to make identification without a time delay. For this lesson, then, only two instruments will be used. It is also assumed that the listener has been able to "remember" the sound for a count of up to seven after the instrument has been sounded.

1. With the listener seated comfortably across the table from you, sound each instrument and allow him to sound each instrument in turn. Encourage him to remember how each sounds. Tell about the fact that they sound almost the same but discuss the sound differences involved.
2. Ask the listener to put his head down on the table and keep it down until you tap him on the shoulder and say, "ready." Explain that you will sound only one of the bells but that you will count (silently) up to ten before you ask him to tell you which it was.
3. Repeat the above exercise, but this time, count *aloud* to ten for the time lapse. If the counting aloud interferes with success, try again and count only to five, then gradually increase the count.

Teacher's Comments:

Checklist:

——— 1. Seems to understand by discussion that although the bells look somewhat alike and sound somewhat alike, there are certain differences in the way they sound.

——— 2. Can remember and identify which of two sound instruments was sounded when the teacher counts silently to ten before requesting identification.

——— 3. Can remember and identify which of two instruments was sounded when the teacher counts to ten aloud before requesting identification of the instrument.

Step V.

It is necessary to remember and identify not only the sounds and their acoustic properties but also the ordinal arrangement in which sounds occur. This ordinal arrangement is called Sound Sequencing. A young child can more readily remember and identify the order in which two or more nonspeech sounds occurred than with speech sounds. Again, the importance of preparing the auditorially disabled person with this background of skill based on gross instrument sounds is emphasized.

Many of the auditorially disabled childen will begin to falter with exercises dealing with auditory memory and sequencing of sound. It is important, therefore, to present these lessons in small, carefully constructed steps. Lessons should be carefully graduated in terms of difficulty in such small increments that the listener is almost sure to succeed.

A. Using two instruments, demonstrate to the listener that he will be listening for *two* sounds this time. This should be through the auditory training unit at a comfortably loud volume. The listener must identify the sounds in the correct sequence.

B. Add a third instrument and repeat the above exercise. Gradually increase the number of instruments to five. You will still sound only *two*.

C. Vary the instruments from time to time, adding new ones in order to assure that the listening skill is progressing upward.

D. Revert to three instruments. Sound all three and ask the listener to resound them or identify them in the correct sequence.

E. Increase the number of choices to five or beyond for identification of a sequence of three instruments to be sounded.

F. Introduce the concept of localization. Sound two instruments in different parts of the room. In response, the child may point to the direction from which the first sound came and then to the direction from which the second sound came.

G. Repeat the above exercises with gradually decreasing volume.
H. Repeat the above exercises, using prerecorded sounds.
I. Repeat all exercises, introducing a gradually increasing time lapse to develop *auditory memory*.
J. Repeat all above procedures against background noise which is gradually increased in loudness.

For the Hearing Impaired:

Repeat the above exercises, using the listener's hearing aid at a comfortably loud level. Gradually decrease the volume of the stimulus sounds.

SAMPLE LESSON PLAN FOR MEMORY OF GROSS SOUND SEQUENCE

Objectives:
1. Reinforcement of the listener's auditory memory.
2. Development of the listener's skill in memory for sound sequencing utilizing two unlike sound instruments.

Materials: Eggbeater and toy squeaker

Activity:
1. With the listener seated comfortably across the table from you, demonstrate the procedure he is to follow: he may watch for the demonstration process.
   A. Sound the toy squeaker. Name it. Allow the listener to do the same.
   B. Turn the crank of the eggbeater, Name it. Encourage the listener to do the same.
   C. Call attention to the sound differences.
   D. Sound one instrument. Identify it. Repeat but ask listener to identify it.
   E. Explain that this time you will sound both instruments and you will have to remember which came first and which came second. Do it yourself first. Encourage the listener to perform the task.
2. Request the listener to turn his head so that vision is obscured. Sound one instrument, then the other. Ask the listener to identify which was

heard first and which second. Repeat procedure, mixing the presentation in order to avoid "patterning."

3. Reverse roles in order to give the listener further insight into the process of sound sequencing.

Teacher's Comments

Checklist:

——— 1. Understands how he is to respond after teacher demonstrates.

——— 2. Recognizes differences between the two sound instruments.

——— 3. Correctly identifies order in which two sound instruments are presented. (Vision obscured)

——— 4. Can successfully assume role of teacher when roles are reversed.

Step VI. *Memory for Sound Sequencing and Projected Listening Utilizing Rhythm*

A. Seated across the table from the listener, repeat the comfortably loud sequence of two instruments as a review procedure. Now move a short distance away from the listener to force him to project his listening in terms of physical distance.

B. Gradually increase the number of instruments to five or more.

C. Increase the number of instruments to be sounded *in sequence* to three.

D. Introduce localization of the above instruments.

E. Repeat above procedures with gradually decreasing volume.

F. Using a drum, or by clapping your hands, present one, two, or three taps. Ask the listener to reproduce the correct number of sounds heard.

G. Present sounds in varying rhythm. For example
one-two - - - - pause - - - - three-four,
one - - - - pause - - - - two-three,
etc. The listener should reproduce the rhythm

H. Repeat the above step (G) and introduce the elements of loudness and softness into the rhythm.
I. Repeat the above exercises using prerecorded sounds.
J. Repeat all exercises, introducing a time lapse for development of auditory memory.
K. Repeat above exercises against gradually increasing background sound. A radio, television, or tape recorder may be utilized here.

For The Hearing Impaired:
A. Present exercises, using the listener's hearing aid.
B. Gradually increase the distance to as far a point as possible.
C. Present above exercises with gradually reduced volume.

SAMPLE LESSON PLAN FOR SOUND SEQUENCING AND PROJECTED LISTENING UTILIZING RHYTHM

Objectives:
1. Reinforcement of the listener's skill in retaining the order for sound sequence.
2. The listener will accomplish objective number one with distance as an added difficulty factor.
3. Development of skill in recognizing and reproducing rhythm.

Materials: Drum. (This may be a coffee can with plastic lid. The outside of can may be decorated.)

Activity: Demonstrate the procedure and manner in which listener is expected to respond. Allow him to observe visually the first time, then he should respond with vision obscured.
1. Present one or two taps on the drum. Listener should reproduce. Gradually increase the number of taps to three or more.
2. Introduce pauses in order to obtain a rhythm which, along with the correct number of taps should be reproduced.

   Example: One pause two,
   One two,
   One two pause three,
   One pause two three,
   etc.

Teacher's
Comments:

Checklist:

——— 1. Can reproduce one or two taps after watching.
——— 2. Can reproduce one or two taps with vision obscured.
——— 3. Can reproduce up to three taps with vision obscured.
——— 4. Can reproduce four taps with vision obscured.
——— 5. Can reproduce up to three taps with pauses introduced for rhythm.
——— 6. Can reproduce up to four taps with pauses, creating rhythm.
——— 7. Can reproduce more than four taps involving pauses for rhythm.

Step VII. *Exercises for Discriminating Pitch and Loudness*

A. Assist the listener to discriminate and identify "high" and "low" pitched tones on the piano, vocal production, tapping of glasses, pans, boxes, etc., which represent high or low tones.
B. Assist the listener to discriminate and identify loud and soft sounds.
C. Repeat all exercises, gradually introducing more nearly similar sounds.
D. Repeat all exercises, introducing gradually increasing background noise, as explained in prior lesson.
E. Repeat above exercises, utilizing prerecorded sound.

Step VIII. *Skills in Auditory Blending*

Auditory blending is a logical exercise to follow auditory memory and auditory sequencing. Blending of two or more sound sources into a more nearly single sound production is sometimes a difficult task for the auditorially disabled person. Begin with one or two gross instruments sounded separately and assist the listener toward sounding them more nearly together without long time delays between.

Step IX. *Skills in Auditory Closure*

Auditory Closure is recognizing and correctly reproducing a word when one or more of the sounds are omitted.

Assist the listener to develop auditory closure skill as follows:

1. Present three instruments. Sound two. Ask the listener which instrument was omitted. He may watch procedures for this demonstration.
2. Repeat the exercise with the listener's vision obscured.
3. Increase the number of instruments to be used to four or more.
4. Repeat above steps with two omissions.

Note: This completes the sequence for developing skills in listening for and identifying *gross sounds.* However, it may be profitable to devote a few moments of each auditory training session to brief review in this area as a "warm up" exercise.

CHAPTER V

AUDITORY PERCEPTUAL EXERCISES USING ANIMAL SOUNDS: A TRANSITIONAL STEP TO SPEECH SOUNDS

As the infant develops awareness and a degree of discrimination for gross sounds, he progresses through the stage of babbling, a well-known developmental speech and language landmark which emerges at approximately six months of age. During this period, the young infant probably produces more sounds than are utilized in the English language. The reason that the child stops using these extra-English sounds is that he begins to listen more selectively to the sounds of the "significant others" in his environment, who fail to reinforce them. Following the babbling period, the child begins a kind of repititious production of syllables, along with babbling. These syllable sounds are refined into word-like sounds and finally, at about age one year, into true, simple words.

In order to avoid confusion on the part of the auditorially disabled individual, live animal sounds should be introduced first. A visit to a farm or zoo will permit the listener to hear live animal sound production. Attention should be directed toward the sounds which individual animals make. The teacher can then imitate these sounds and encourage the listener to do likewise. If such a visit is not possible, a film or slide program with good tape-recorded sound reproductions which can be ascribed to the appropriate animal would be desirable.

Following the experience of hearing the live animal sounds, tape recordings, records, or video tape recordings may be used to reinforce the experience before proceeding to the next step which involves production of animal sounds, using the human voice.

Animal sounds, as they are produced by humans, are composed of one or more consonant sounds plus a vowel. Certain animal sounds are composed of diphthongs (combinations of two vowels) as the *oink*—the sound made by the pig as produced by humans. Animal sounds are in keeping with the developmental model: Human production of animal sounds are speech sounds which are stripped of human personification. In some cases, animal sounds may eliminate the anxiety associated with speech for certain individuals; especially where an emotional overlay complicates his functioning.

Training must progress from gross to fine listening skills.[1]

The transition from gross sound stimuli to animal sounds represents the kind of structuring necessary for certain auditorially disabled individuals.

Step I. *Discrimination For Animal Sounds*

A. At a comfortably loud level, introduce a miniature or picture of a cow. Also on the table, place one or two of the familiar, gross sound instruments. Hold the cow near your lips and say, "The cow says, 'Mooooo'."

B. Gradually replace gross instruments with animal miniatures or pictures until you are working exclusively with animal sounds. Present all new sounds in the same manner as suggested in Step IA. If the listener repeats the sound, do not discourage him.

Suggested Sounds:

Cow .... Moo
Dog .... Bow wow
Sheep .... Ba-a-a

[1] Battin, R. Ray and Haug, C. Olaf: *Speech and Language Delay, A Home Training Program.* Illinois, Charles C Thomas Publisher, 1964, p. 40.

Horse . . . . He-e-e
Bird . . . . Tweet-tweet
Duck . . . . Quack-quack
Chicken . . . . Cluck-cluck
Cat . . . . Meow
Mouse . . . . Eek-eek
Pig . . . . Oink

C. Gradually present many animal sounds until the listener can identify consistently any of three.

D. Assist the listener to *localize* the direction from which the sound came. Place the animals in two locations in the room. Sound one. Request the listener to point to the correct direction, or to verbalize the animal's name. Increase the number of locations to three or more as the listener gains skill.

E. Increase the choices at a given sitting to four animals, then five or more.

F. Repeat the above steps with gradually lowered level of intensity.

Step II. *Improvement of Auditory Memory Span*

A. Repeat the exercises in Step I at normal volume but with a short time lapse. This is to assist the listener to develop auditory memory. Begin with a count of two or three. Gradually increase the count as the listener gains skill.

B. Repeat the task as outlined in Step II-A with gradually reduced volume.

C. Repeat exercises in Step II-A and B. using prerecorded sounds.

For the Hearing Impaired:

1. Repeat all exercises in this part, using the listener's hearing aid as the source of amplification. Gradually reduce the volume as the listener gains skill.
2. Repeat as many steps as possible without amplification.

3. Repeat above exercises against gradually increasing background noise, first with comfortably loud amplification through the hearing aid, then at reduced levels of intensity.

Step III. *Development of Auditory Sequencing Skill*

A. Use two animal sounds. Indicate to the listener that he is to remember which sound was heard first and which sound was heard second. Demonstrate what is expected of him. This presentation should be at a comfortable listening level of loudness.

B. After demonstrating the technique, indicate that it is the listener's turn to make identification. Vision must be obscured. Praise correct identification. If an error is made, demonstrate all sounds again. Encourage the listener to re-auditorize the sounds. Sound one, place the listener's hand on it, and say, "This was *first*." Sound a second animal. Place the listener's hand on the appropriate animal and say, "This was *second*." Repeat the procedure once or twice while the listener watches, then again try with his vision obscured.

C. Add a third, then fourth, then fifth animal sound.

D. Assist the listener to *localize* sound by moving to various parts of the room.
If the listener is hearing impaired, he must wear binaural amplification, or none at all.

E. Repeat above exercises with reduced volume.

F. Repeat above exercises using prerecorded sounds.

G. Gradually move to a farther distance from the listener to force him to project his listening abilities.

H. Repeat the above exercises with emphasis on either high or low sound pitch. The speaker who presents the sound must attempt to maintain consistent voice throughout. The cow, duck, dog, and sheep may represent low-pitched sound. The bird, mouse, and horse may represent high-pitched sound. Arrange for the listener to identify pitch by some appropriate signal such as pointing *up* for high-pitched sound and *down* for low.

I. Repeat the above exercises at reduced levels of loudness.

J. Present the exercises more rapidly.

K. Teach the listener to discriminate for loudness and softness. Gradually reduce the level of intensity at which the stimulus is presented.

L. Repeat the above exercises against gradually louder background sounds.

For the Hearing Impaired:

1. Repeat all of the above exercises using the listener's hearing aid as the means of amplification.
2. Gradually reduce the volume of loudness.
3. Repeat the above exercises without amplification, if possible.
4. Repeat the above exercises with amplification but with gradually increasingly loud background sound.

SAMPLE LESSON PLAN FOR DISCRIMINATION OF ANIMAL SOUNDS

Objective: Discrimination between two unlike animal sounds in the presence of background sound.

Materials:

1. Seated comfortably at a table across from the listener, hold the cat near your lips and say, "the cat says meow." This should be fairly high pitched. Ask the listener to do the same, then request him to place the cat on the table.
2. Repeat the procedure for the sound made by the duck. This should be fairly low in pitch.
3. Obscure the listener's vision, then assist him to make identification of the correct animal whose sound you made.

4. Repeat the above against gradually increasing background sound from the radio or record player.

Teacher's
Comments:

Checklist:

_______ Can correctly identify the sound made by the cat and duck.

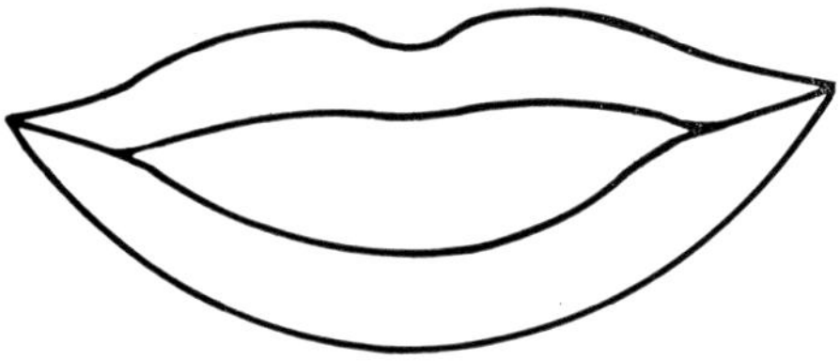

(i) as in feet

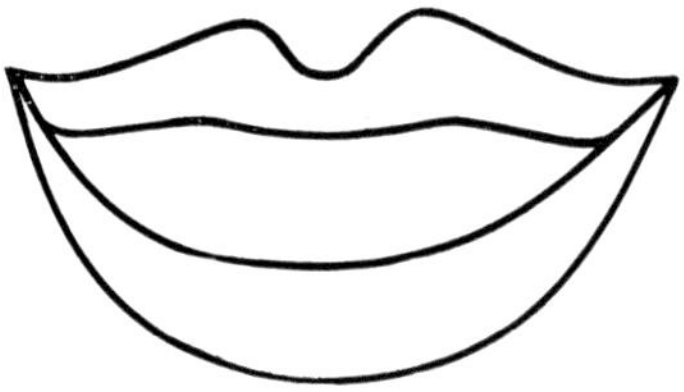

(e) as in late

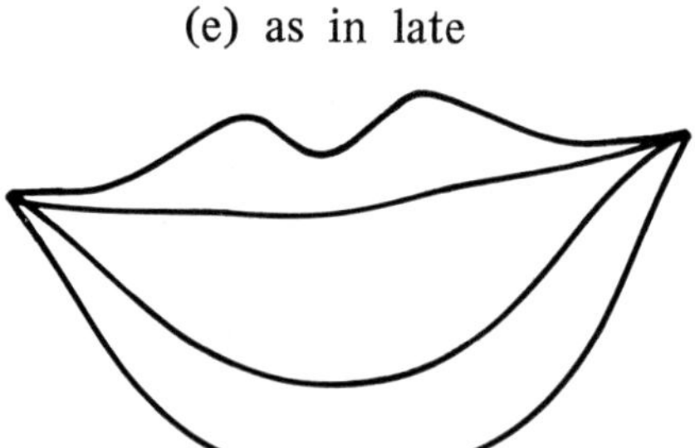

(æ) as in cat

Figure 1.

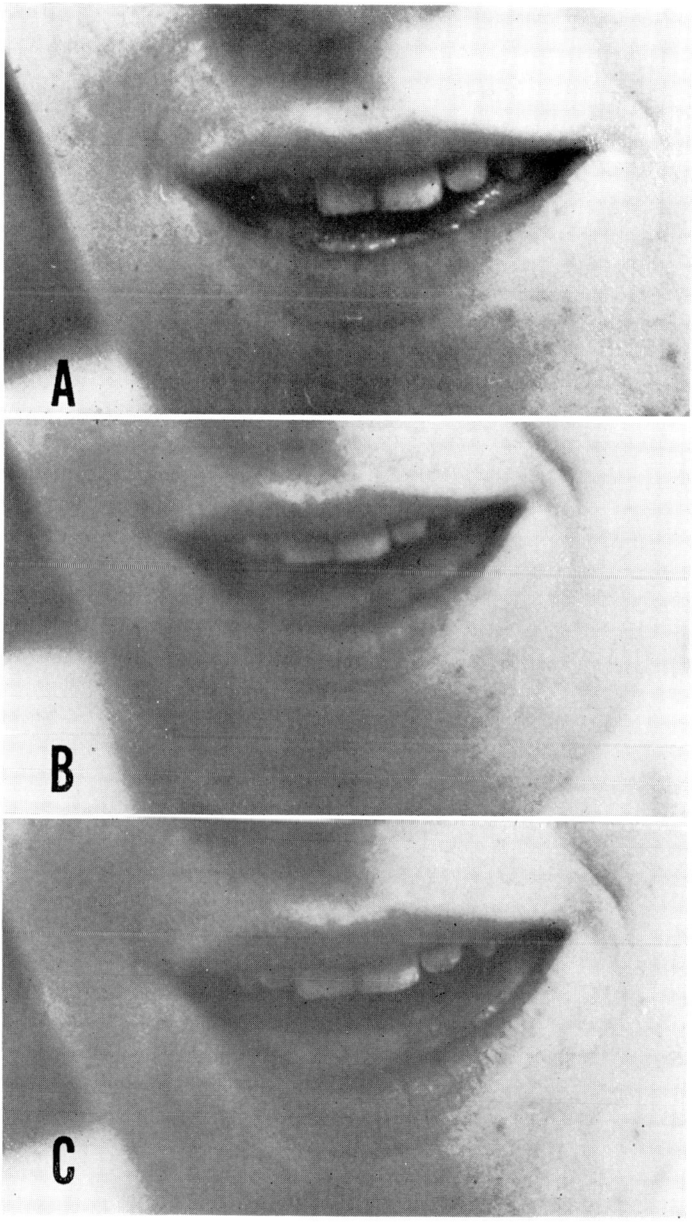

Figure 2. Vowels. A. (i) as in feet; B. (e) as in late; C. (æ) as in cat.

________ Can correctly make the sounds for the cat or duck.

________ Can consistently identify the animal sound when vision is obscured.

________ Can consistently identify the animal sound when soft background sound is present.

________ Can consistently identify the animal sound when background sound is almost as loud as the animal sound for which he listened.

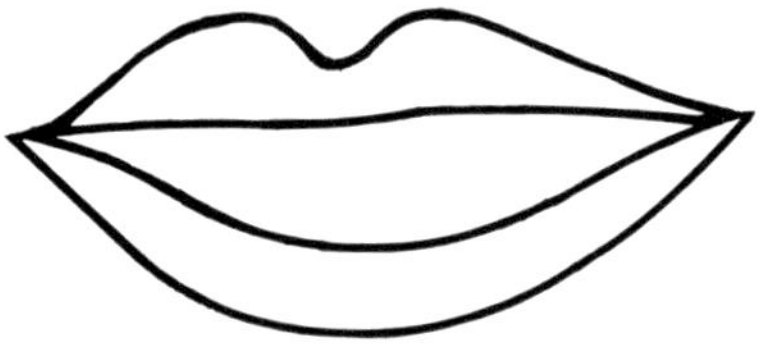

(ɔ) as in ball

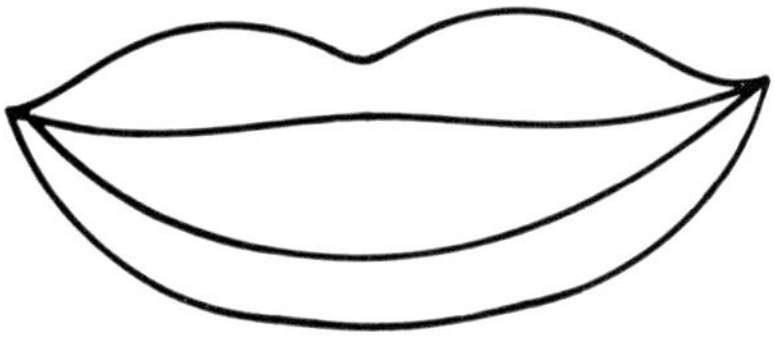

(ʌ) as in cup

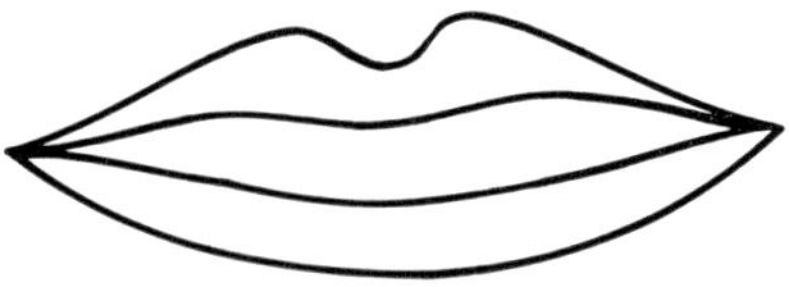

(u) as in book

Figure 3.

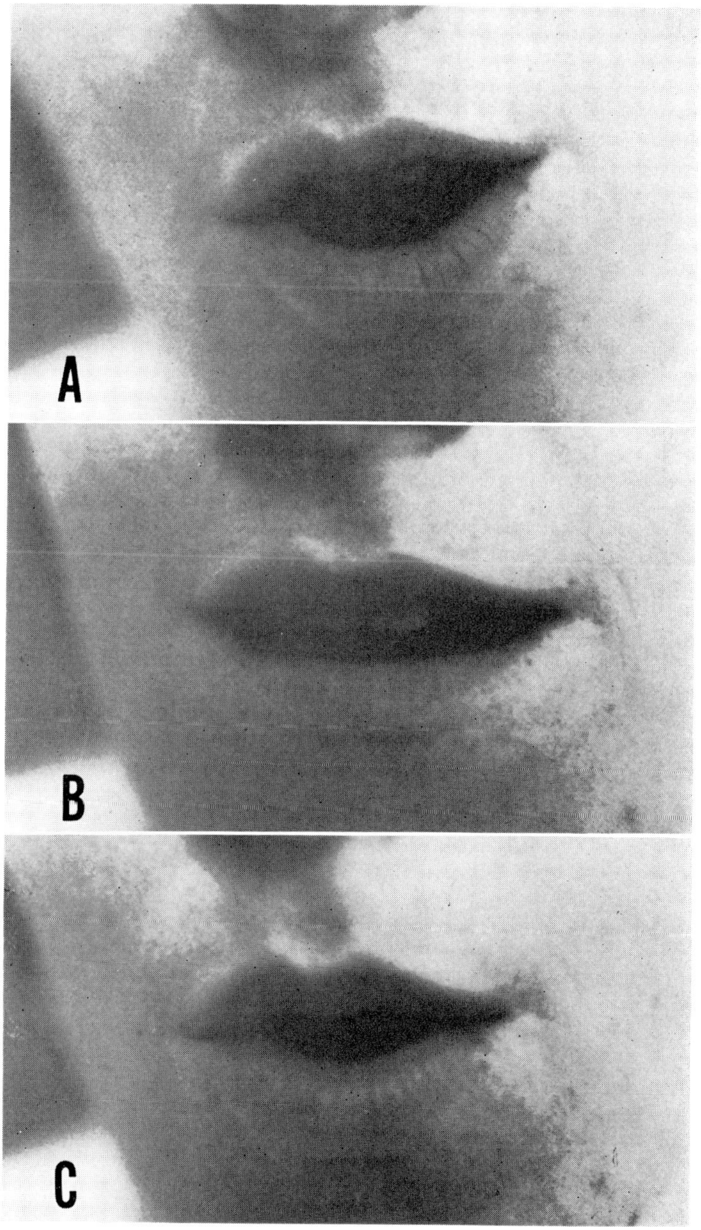

Figure 4. Vowels. A. (ɔ) as in ball; B. (ʌ) as in cup; C. (u) as in book.

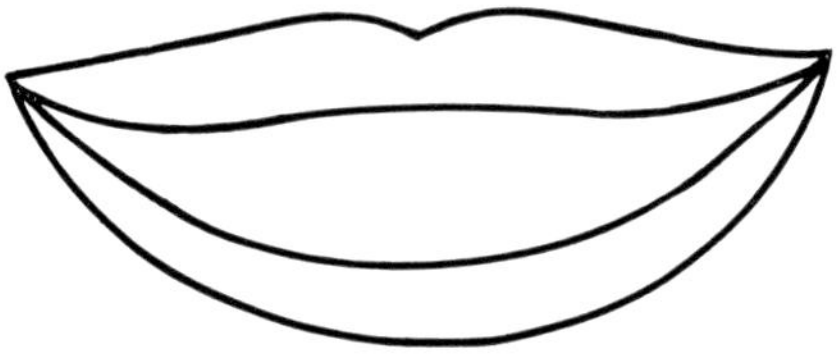

(I) as in sit

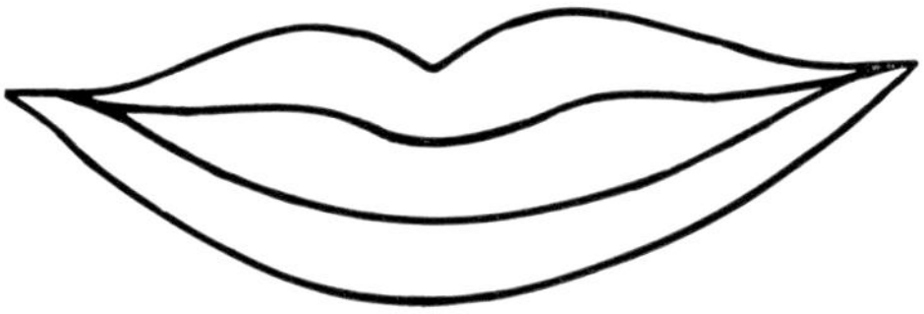

(ɛ) as in hen

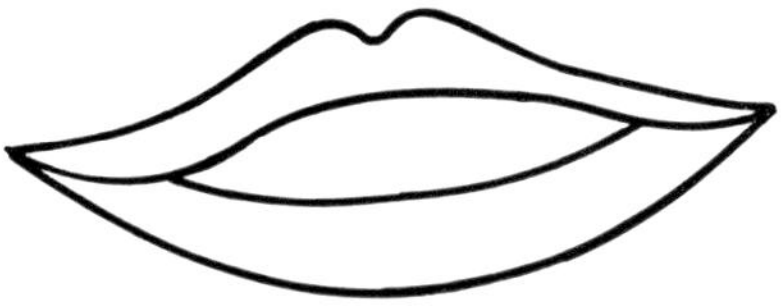

(a) as in father

Figure 5.

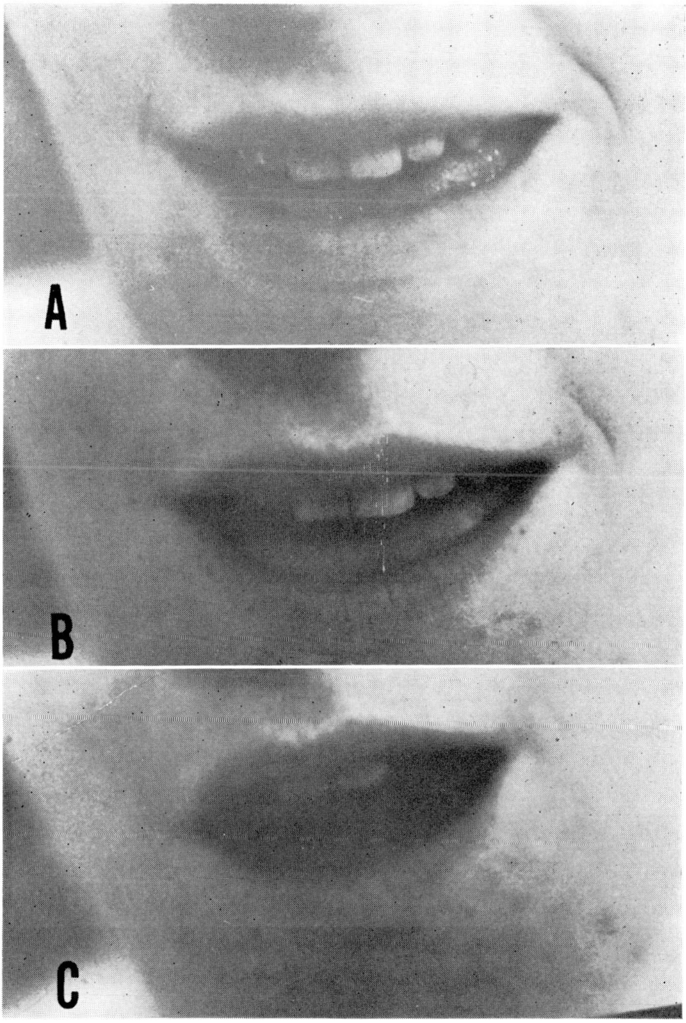

Figure 6. Vowels. A. (I) as in sit; B. (ε) as in hen; C. (a) as in father.

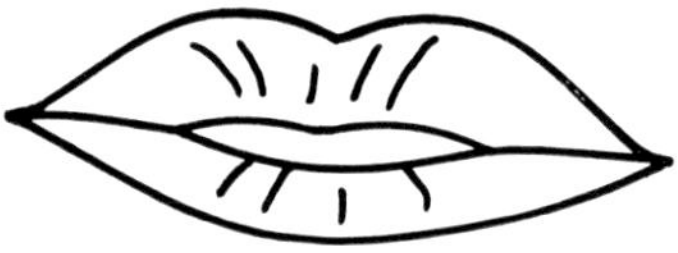

(o) as in boat

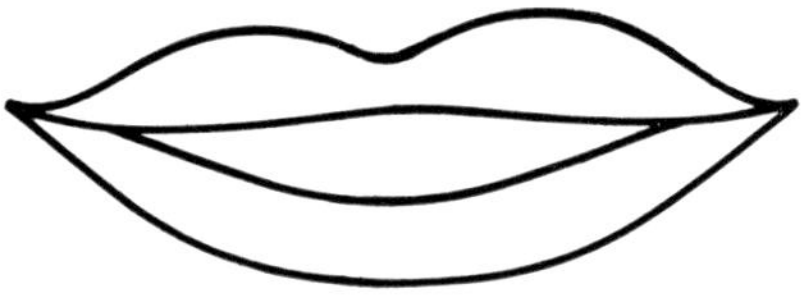

(ɝ) as in bird

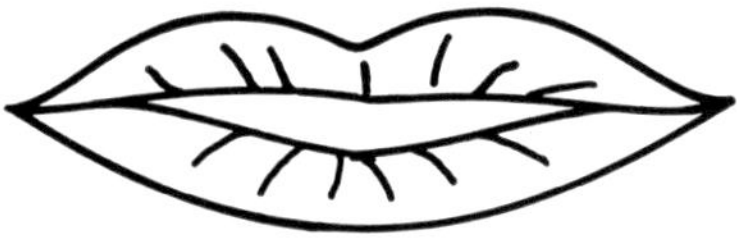

(u) as in boot

Figure 7.

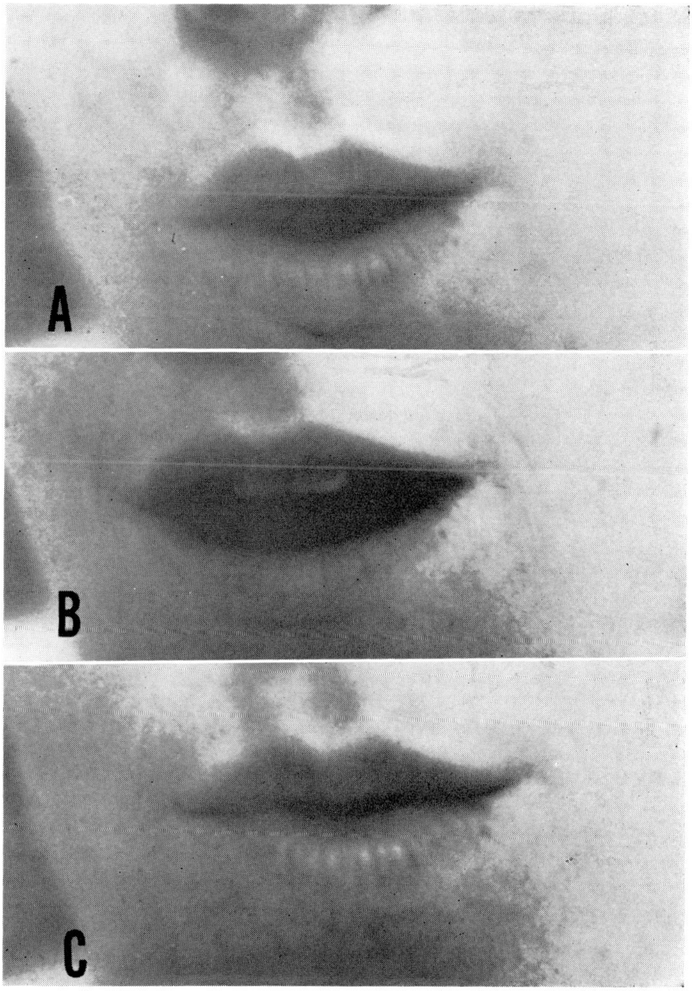

Figure 8. Vowels. A. (o) as in boat; B. (ɝ) as in bird; C. (u) as in boot.

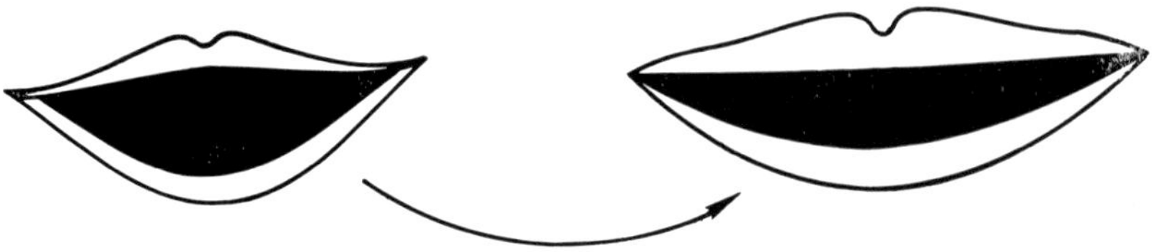

(aI) as in ride

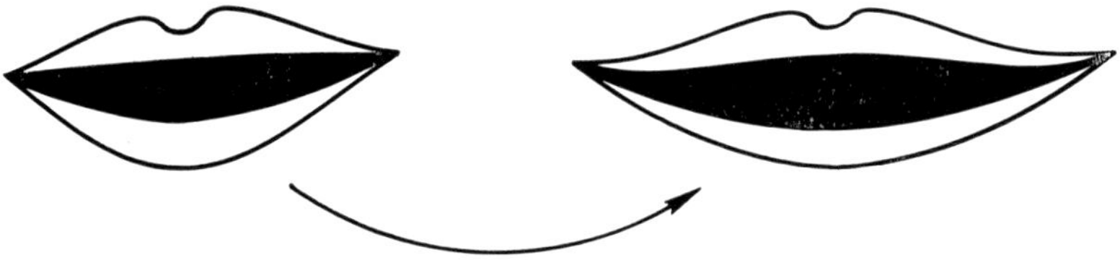

(oI) as in boy

Figure 9. Diphthongs.

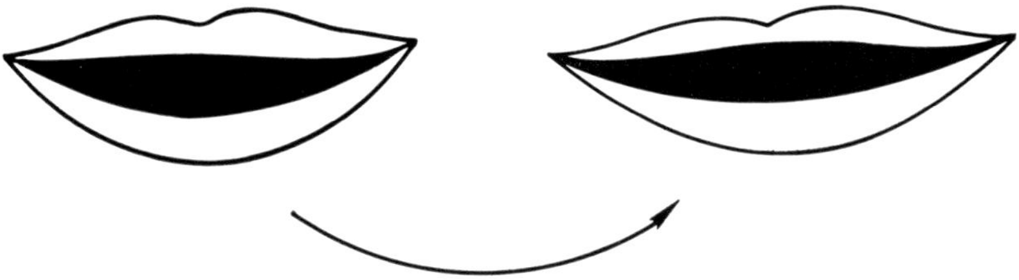

(eI) as in day

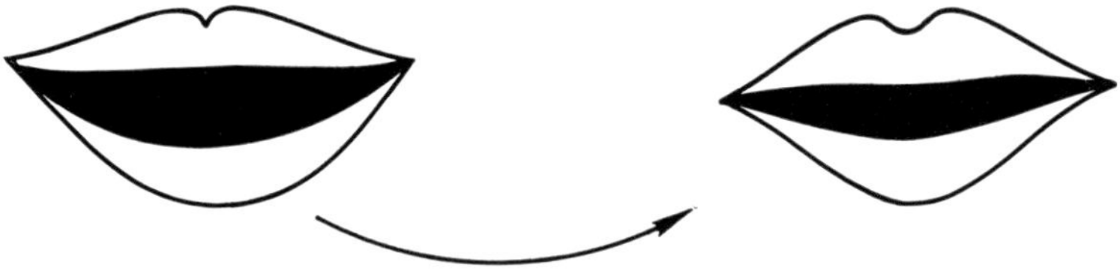

(au) as in cow

Figure 10. Diphthongs.

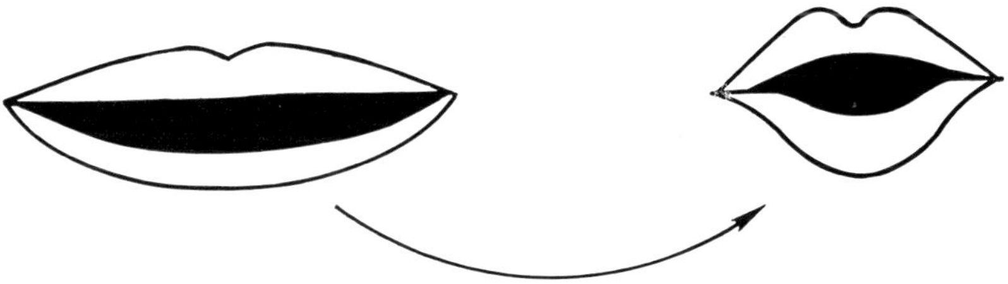

(iu) as in few

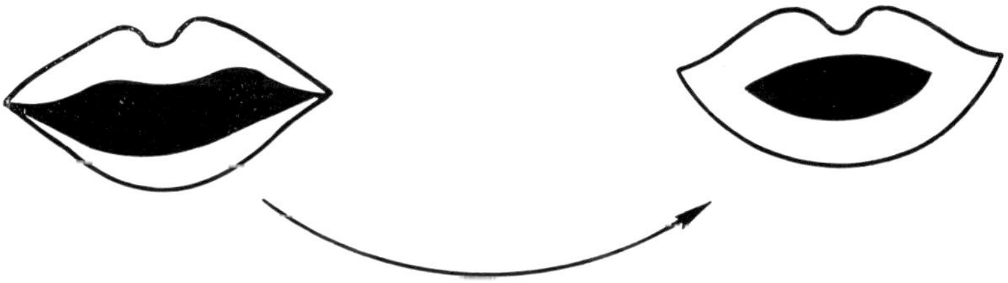

(ou) as in show

Figure 11. Diphthongs.

CHAPTER VI

AUDITORY PERCEPTUAL EXERCISES FOR VOWEL SOUNDS

REFERRING AGAIN to the Developmental Model, the presentation of vowel sounds may be likened to the babbling stage which was discussed briefly in the last chapter and which occurs in the young child at approximately six months of age.

> Although there is no predetermined order of appearance of the various sounds heard in babbling, the liklihood is that the child will produce vowels before consonants. Of the vowels, a variety of (ɑ) repeated at length with variations in pitch and loudness will probably be among the first to be heard.[1]

At this stage, lessons may be based on the listener's own successful productions. The teacher should feed back any spontaneous productions provided by the listener. These sounds may then be incorporated into the lesson.

Research studies have demonstrated that young children attend more easily to a visual line drawing than to actual photographs. In keeping with the normal developmental taxonomy, then, line drawings for vowels precede photographs of lips forming the sounds. In addition, line drawings for several diphthongs are provided.

Step I. *Developing Awareness of Volume Sounds:*

In this exercise, pictures of the vowel sounds on the lips may be used as the basis of the listener's

[1] Berry, Mildred F. and Eisonson, Jon: *Speech Disorders.* New York, Appleton-Century-Crofts, Inc., 1956, p. 20.

identifying responses. Use first the line drawings provided in this chapter. When the listener identifies the sound consistently with the appropriate line drawing, have him match the sound with BOTH the line drawing and the photograph of a given sound. Eliminate the line drawing and use only the photograph as the listener shows himself capable through consistent, appropriate responses.

At first, present various un*like* vowel and diphthong sounds at a comfortably loud level. Although diphthongs represent a combination of two vowel sounds, they will be presented in the vowel section.

Step II. *Discrimination for Vowel Sounds*

A. Present one of two vowel sounds. Request the listener to identify by pointing to the appropriate picture. This first attempt should be done with the listener watching the lips.

B. The speaker should obscure his lips and repeat Step II-A.

C. Gradually increase the number of pictures to three, then four, five, or more as the listener gains skill.

D. Continue until the listener can identify all of the vowel or diphthong pictures.

E. Repeat the above exercises with lowered volume.

Step III. *Auditory Memory Exercises for Vowels and Diphthongs*

A. Present two volume sounds and require the listener to identify them in the correct sequence. Volume may be comfortably loud.

B. Gradually increase the number of vowels to five or more.

C. Gradually increase the number of sequential vowels to be identified to three.

D. Gradually decrease the volume.

E. Increase the volume and move away from the microphone to assist the listener to project his listening ability.

F. Decrease the volume and repeat the above exercise.

For the Hearing Impaired:

1. Repeat exercises in this step, using the listener's hearing aid as the source of amplification.
2. Repeat the above exercises but introduce background sound.
3. Repeat the above exercises without amplification.
4. Introduce a short time lapse for sequential sounds and repeat above exercises. Gradually extend the time lapse.

Step IV. *Localization of Vowel Sounds*

A. Station two or three persons in various parts of the room. If the teacher must present the lesson without assistance, she should move quietly from one part of the room to the other when she wishes to change directions. Present a vowel sound at a comfortable level of loudness. The listener's back should be turned toward the speaker. The listener can respond by pointing to the correct direction.

B. Repeat the above task with lowered volume.

C. Repeat the above tasks against gradually increasing background sound.

Step V. *Sequencing of Vowel and Diphthong Sounds*

A. Present two vowel sounds and their pictures—Demonstrate the procedure before asking the listener to respond. Sound one vowel, then the other. Touch the first vowel and say, "This was first." Touch the second and say, "This was second. Now it's your turn."

B. Repeat the procedure with the listener watching. Assist him to make the correct choice.

C. Obscure the listener's vision and repeat Step V-A.

D. Gradually increase the number of vowel sounds and their pictures. When the listener has gained some skill, increase the number of sounds to three.

E. Gradually reduce the volume and repeat the above exercises.

F. Introduce a gradually increasing time lapse.

G. Repeat the above exercises with gradually increasing background sound.

For the Hearing Impaired:

1. Present exercises with the hearing aid turned at a comfortably loud level.
2. Gradually lower the volume.
3. Repeat exercises without amplification, if possible.

Step VI. *Development of Projected Listening of Vowels and Diphthongs.*

A. Gradually move farther away from the listener. Request him to identify one of two vowel sounds, then one of three. Continue to increase the number until he can identify one of several choices for vowel sounds.

B. Repeat the above exercise with lowered volume.

C. Introduce a gradually increasing time lapse to assist the listener in developing auditory memory.

D. Introduce gradually louder background sound.

E. Present the above tasks which have been prerecorded.

Step VII. *Discrimination for Pitch of Vowels and Diphthongs.*

A. Develop discrimination for pitch of vowels and diphthongs, by presenting a given sound at either high or low pitch. The individual may make identification by pointing either upward and downward, or saying "high" or "low."

B. Using any two vowels or diphthongs and their accompanying pictures, develop discrimination for *high and low sounds.* This should assist the listener in his production of sound, since vowels and diphthongs can be classified according to the high, low, or medial oral ports of production.

Step VIII. *Discrimination for Volume Sounds*

A. Using any single vowel sound or group of vowels, develop discrimination for loudness and softness by first having the listener identify (respond) by saying "loud" and "soft." By pointing to the written words, or by any appropriate pre-arranged gesture or signal.

B. When the individual can discriminate loudness or softness between two discrete vowel sounds or series of vowel sounds, increase the difficulty by prolonging your voice production and alternating between loudness and softness. The individual should now quickly identify loud and soft as you vocalize.

Step IX. *Developing an awareness of Rhythm in Vowel Sounds*

A. This may be accomplished by using either the same or different vowel sounds. As you vocalize two vowels, emphasize one more than the other. EX: Eē ōh. Teach the listener to express the rhythm by clapping out the pattern of emphasis.

B. To provide a concrete method of response, provide cards in which large and small patterns represent loud and soft sounds.

Example

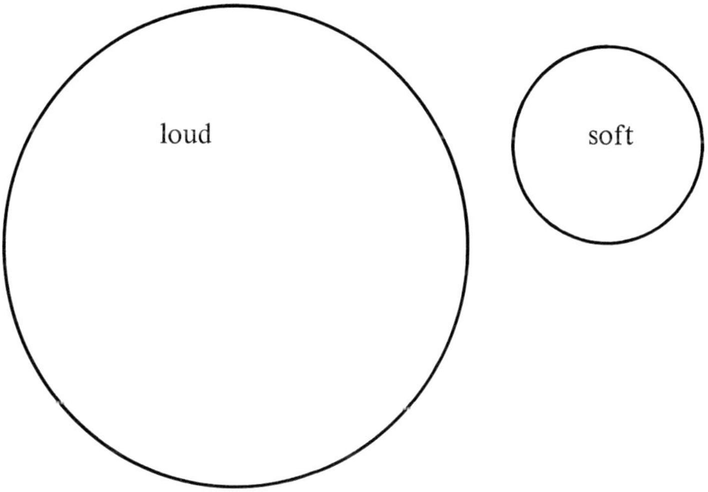

SAMPLE LESSON PLAN FOR AUDITORY PERCEPTION OF VOWELS AND DIPHTHONGS

Objective: The listener will identify in correct sequence two of three vowel sounds.

Materials: Pictures of lip formations for a as in cat
e as in feet
o as in boat

Procedure:

1. The listener will have correctly identified all sound to be used in the lesson. He will have successfully identified the picture related to each sound. The listener will have correctly identified two in the correct sequence from among a choice of the above three pictures.
2. Hold each picture near your lips and give its vowel sound.
3. Demonstrate to the listener how he is expected to respond.

4. Sound the above three vowels in sequence. Allow the listener to watch the procedure. Assist him to make the correct identification.
5. Repeat the above task with the listener's vision obscured.
6. Vary the presentations.

Teacher Comments:

Checklist:

______ Can correctly identify the vowel relating to all of the above pictures.

______ Can correctly identify the sequence of three after watching the teacher make the sounds.

______ Can correctly identify the sequence of three with vision obscured.

______ Can correctly identify any sequence of three with vision obscured.

CHAPTER VII

AUDITORY PERCEPTUAL REMEDIATION BASED ON SPEECH SYLLABLES

The production of speech syllables (a consonant and vowel combination) develops in the normal child by the end of his first year. Much of these productions are simply echoing behavior and at first have no meaning. By one year of age, the child has acquired approximately ten vowels and nine consonants in his babbling, echoing, and lalling behavior.[1]

The manner in which the young child progresses from gross auditory perception to perception and production of vowel sounds then to syllables, is orderly. The production of syllable sounds precedes the first true words. There is much overlapping of the processes. In fact, many syllables are also words. For example: see, saw, me, my, etc.

Step I. *Developing Awareness and Discrimination for Speech Syllables*

A. Syllables should at first involve all initial plosive (b) consonants. Examples: Bee, bow, bah, buy, etc. Use all possible combinations with the initial consonant (b). These syllables may be written on cards for purposes of identification. For the very young child,

[1] Battin, R. Ray and Haug, C. Olaf: *Speech and Language Delay, A Home Training Program*. Illinois, Charles C Thomas Publisher, 1964, p. 8, Fig. 1.

this is more easily accomplished by having the child point to the shape of lips for the appropriate vowel involved, or by having him imitate your production.

B. Add other initial consonants. At first present those which are easily visible on the lips. Examples: m p l d n f and v.

C. Use syllables with the consonants appearing in the final position, such as oop, ape, oap, etc.

Step II. Present the above exercise with a *gradual reduction in loudness.*

Step III. Present the above exercises and introduce the gradually increasing time lapse for development of *auditory memory span for syllables.*

Step IV. Gradually increase the number of syllables at a given sitting to five. You may increase the level of loudness at first, until the listener gains more skill, then it should be again, reduced gradually.

Step V. Repeat all of the above exercises, using *pre-recorded materials* which are repeated in the same way. If it is convenient, you may record your exercises as they are presented to the listener, and use these for future work.

Step VI. Repeat all above exercises, but now *present two sounds in sequence.* The listener must identify them correctly and in correct sequence. He may repeat the sounds, or point to cards with the written syllables appearing on them.

Step VII. Gradually move the listener a short distance away from the microphone so he must *project his listening,* in order to identify the syllables.

For the Hearing Impaired:

Repeat all of above exercises, using the individual's own hearing aid as the source of amplification.

Step VIII. Assist the listener to develop ability to *localize sounds,* using speech syllables. This will require two or three persons stationed at different points in the room. One will vocalize a pre-determined syllable. The child must discriminate the sound as well as the *source* of sound. Reduce the level of loudness, gradually.

Step IX. Help the listener develop *discrimination for pitch,* using syllable sounds. You may use the same syllables throughout, for this exercise, or vary them after the listener gains some skill.

Step X. *Discrimination For Volume of Syllables*

A. Using any single syllable, or group of syllables, assist the listener to discriminate between loudness and softness. At first he can respond by saying "loud" or "soft," or he can point to a large circle to represent *loud* and a small circle (or other figure) to represent *soft.*

B. When the listener can easily and consistently identify loudness and softness, make the signals more nearly alike. They must, however, be identifiable by sufficient differences in volume.

C. As the listener gains skill, speed up the operation.

Step XI. *Developing an awareness for Rhythm in Speech Syllables:*

A. This may be accomplished by using the same syllables or different syllables. As you vocalize two syllables, emphasize one more than the other. Example: Bee-BOW. Teach the listener to express the rhythm by clapping out the pattern of emphasis.

B. If necessary, provide a visual clue consisting of a large circle for emphasis, and a small circle for non-emphasis.

Step XII. *Discrimination for Pitch of Speech Syllables:*

A. Assist the listener to develop discrimination for pitch of speech syllables by presenting either a high or low pitched production. The individual should make identification by pointing upward for *high* or downward for *low.*

B. As the listener gains skill, have him verbalize his identification of "high" or "low."

C. Speed up the production-identification process as the listener shows capability.

D. Reverse roles after the listener has gained sufficient skill and confidence.

Step XIII. *Discrimination For Syllables Against Background Sound.*

A. Repeat any of the materials presented thus far in syllable work. Introduce a very soft background sound. Explain to the listener that he is to ignore the background sound and listen only to the syllables so he can identify them correctly. Explain the importance of paying attention to lesson materials and not attending to other (extraneous) sounds.

B. Gradually increase the volume of the background sound.

C. Repeat the above exercises and introduce a gradually increasing time lapse in order to develop memory for syllables against an interfering sound signal.

For the Hearing Impaired:

1. Use binaural hearing aids for localization.
2. Repeat above exercises with reduced amplification to the extent that it is possible.

SAMPLE LESSON PLAN FOR DISCRIMINATION OF SPEECH SYLLABLES

Objectives: 1. To assist the listener to improve awareness for speech syllables.

2. To assist the listener to improve ability to discriminate speech syllables with the consonant in either the initial or final position.

Materials: 3 x 5 cards on each of which is written one of the following syllables. BEE BOW BUY AHB EEB OWB.

Activity: With the listener seated comfortably across the table from you, demonstrate the procedure he is to follow. He should be permitted to watch the demonstration lesson, after which his vision should be obscured for subsequent operations.

1. Verbalize the syllables, holding the appropriate card near your lips as you do so. Use only the cards having the initial consonant.
2. Pretend to obscure your vision (by closing your eyes, putting your head down, or by holding a card in front of your eyes) then sound one syllable.
3. Tap yourself on the arm and say, "Ready!" Look at all three cards then point to the correct one.
4. Assist the listener to perform the task. Present any and all of the syllables on the cards.
5. Present, in the same way, the syllables with the final consonant sounds.
6. Repeat the above exercises with consonant sounds in either initial or final positions.

Teacher's Comments:

Checklist:

______ 1. Can identify any one of three syllables with the initial consonant sound.

______ 2. Can identify any one of three syllables with the final consonant sound.

______ 3. Can identify four of any six syllables with the consonant sounds in unstructured order.

CHAPTER VIII

AUDITORY PERCEPTUAL REMEDIATION: WORD BASED

THE ULTIMATE PURPOSE of auditory perceptual training is to assist the auditorially disabled individual establish adequate verbal language communication. Complex listening skills precede emergence of the babbling stage of the infant. Auditorially, he must have reached this language landmark before he could perform even the basic listening tasks outlined in this book. At the babbling stage, the child enjoys the sound of his own vocal productions and he is, therefore, at least aware of sound.

The speech syllable lessons in this book may be likened to the echolalia and lalling stages through which the child progresses at approximately eight to twelve months of age.

Lessons based on single words at the naming level, may be compared to the naming activities of the child at approximately one to two years of age. The "significant others" in the listener's environment should stimulate him with commonly used nouns, verbs, and prepositions which may easily be utilized in these lessons. Such stimulation will also improve the listener's vocabulary.

It would be desirable, at this level, to adapt a basic language development program into the daily lessons, if the listener's language deprivation warrants it. A program such as Heasley's Basic Language Development Program (unpublished as of November, 1972) would be appropriate.[1] Also, the Assessment of Children's Language Comprehension (ACLC)[2] is a simple measure of the

[1] Heasley, Bernice E.: *A Basic Language Development Program.* Unpub.

[2] Foster, Rochana, Giddan, Jane J., and Stark, Joel: *Assessment of Children's Language Comprehension.* Consulting Psychologists Press, Inc., 1972.

level at which the individual is functioning language-wise. The vocabulary is recycled for all levels of difficulty. This inventory provides information about the kinds of language which the listener can process. It identifies the level at which remediation should begin.

These lessons are based upon the traditional speech correction model. That is, words involve a given consonant sound first in the initial position, then in the final position, and finally, in the more difficult medial position. Lessons are developed in the carefully structured steps employed by speech correctionists.

DISCRIMINATION FOR WORDS

Step I. A. As a transitional step from syllables to words, the first words may involve only a single syllable. The teacher should compile a list of simple words which are useful to the individual. First words should be composed of a single consonant in the initial position. Below is a suggested list of words for the consonant (b):

ball	barn	box
bee	bell	bite
Bye (buy)	boat	big
bat	book	blue
boy	bed	bowl
bear	belt	bite

B. Next present words with (b) in the final position, then in the medial position.

Final Position	*Medial Position*
tub	able
rub	baby
rob	rabbit
robe	table
bib	about

C. Present one of two words for the listener to identify. Increase the number of word presentations as the listener demonstrates skill by appropriate, consistent responses.

D. When the listener has acquired sufficient skill in identifying words in which (b) occurs in the initial, final, and medial positions, the teacher can begin to present words which incorporate other consonants which are easily visible when they are produced. Such sounds as p, m, n, l, d, t, f, and v would be appropriate. The teacher should compile word lists for each of these sounds. The words should be core vocabulary words. The list should include words in which the specific sound occurs in all positions; that is, the initial, medial and final.

When approximately 75% success in identification has been achieved with words in which the consonant sound is easily visible, the teacher may begin to present words which incorporate consonants which are less visible on the lips when they are produced. For example, k, s, g, ng, r, sh, etc. are less visible.

The teacher should present a choice of two words when she introduces a new sound. This can be increased to three as the listener gains skill. These should be presented at a comfortable level of intensity. The volume should be decreased as the listener gains skill.

E. Increase the rate of presentation as the listener demonstrates skill.

F. Gradually introduce soft background sound which the listener should be assisted to ignore. This may be provided by a radio, television, tape recorder, or by the teacher shuffling feet, moving books, and similar tactics. If it is a group lesson, the group can be instructed to provide background sound when the teacher gives them a signal.

The background should be gradually increased in intensity as the listener gains skill.

Step II. Repeat the above exercises at a gradually reduced level of loudness to force the listener's attending ability.

Step III. Repeat the above exercises, introducing a gradually increasing time lapse to assist the auditorially disabled individual to develop auditory memory span.

Step IV. Gradually increase the number of words at a given sitting to five. Increase the level of loudness to a comfortable level each time you increase the number. Gradually reduce the volume when the listener can identify the words fairly consistently.

Step V. Try to develop the ability to localize sound, using words.

Step VI. Repeat all of the above steps in this part, but require identification of two words in correct sequence. Increase the volume of presentation slightly at first, then decrease it as quickly as listener skill permits.

Step VII. Gradually move a short distance away from the individual. This forces him to project his listening in terms of physical distance.

Step VIII. Repeat all of the above steps at a gradually increased distance.

Step IX. Present the above exercises in tape recorded form. Assist the listener to attend to the recording and follow instructions as given. Be sure that the lessons are simple, familiar, and explicit as to content and method of listener response. Gradually reduce the volume of the recorder for the same and for similar lessons.

Step X. Develop discrimination for pitch, using words. You may use either the same or different words for this exercise. As the listener gains skill, however, it would be useful to encourage him to listen for and identify the words as well as pitch.

Step XI. Repeat the above exercise, with gradually reduced volume.

Step XII. Develop discrimination for loudness-softness, using words. The number of syllables per word may vary. This may be developed by the same procedures followed in developing discrimination in vowels and syllables.

Step XIII. Assist the listener to develop *discrimination for Rhythm of Words* in the same manner in which you presented rhythm for vowels and syllables.

Step XIV. Repeat all exercises in this part, using SIMILAR WORDS.

Examples:		
	rain	main
	bear	pear
	able	table
	king	ring
	Sunday	Monday

Step XV. Develop an *Awareness for Inflection of Words*, using the same procedures as those used to develop awareness for inflection of vowel sounds and syllables.

For the Hearing Impaired:

1. Present lessons at a comfortable level of loudness, then gradually reduce the volume of sound.
2. The localization exercise will require either binaural amplification, or no amplification at all. This will require two or three persons stationed at various points in the room. One will say a word. The listener will point in the proper direction. The listener's vision should be obscured for this exercise.

SAMPLE LESSON PLAN DISCRIMINATION OF PITCH IN WORDS

Objective: The listener will discriminate high or low pitch in word presentations.

Materials: A short list of words which can easily be presented at either high or low pitch. A few words are suggested below:

yes no why oh hi who? where? when? stop

Activity: This lesson assumes prior skill in identifying high and low pitch in vowels and syllables. It assumed that the listener understand the method by which he will make pitch identification. This may be by means of pointing up for high and down for low, or by saying "high" or "low."

1. Present three words at high pitch. Assist the listener to identify them correctly.
   Present three words at low pitch. Assist the listener to identify them correctly.
2. Present the same three words at either high or low pitch. Assist the listener to identify them correctly.
3. Increase the number of words in any given presentation.
4. Reverse roles.

Teacher's Comments:

Checklist:

_______ 1. Can identify the correct pitch of any one of three words which are presented at a high pitch.

_______ 2. Can identify correctly the pitch for any one of the same three words which are presented at low pitch.

_______ 3. Can correctly identify the pitch for any of the same three words when the pitch is presented in random order.

_______ 4. Can reverse roles for steps 1 and 2.

_______ 5. Can reverse roles for step 3.

CHAPTER IX

AUDITORY PERCEPTUAL REMEDIATION BASED ON CONNECTED SPEECH

In the developing child, the first "true words" lead to fairly rapid language acquisition and expression of one-word sentences. That is, a single word is intended to symbolize a fairly complete thought. As an example, "Coat" becomes "Get coat" or "Where coat?" to "Where Bobby's coat?" to "Where my coat?" and finally, "Where is my coat?"

At the connected speech level, it is reasonable to assume that the listener brings a degree of language acquisition to the lesson situation even though he may perceive or process some or all of the signals in a subnormal way. Lessons at this level, then, may begin with discrimination tasks, omitting the awareness factor. At this level, the auditorially disabled individual is likely to demonstrate difficulty with memory tasks which involve sequencing, blending, and closure components. Butler has stated that "auditory sequential memory may be the best predictor of school achievement over all the academic subjects tested (i.e. reading, spelling, and arithmetic.) [1]

Connected speech involves all of the individual components associated with auditory processing. It is for this reason that auditorially disabled persons use individual words appropriately but fail to connect them into meaningful verbal language. The

[1] Butler, Katharine G.: *A Focus on Current Research in Auditory Perception.* Proceedings of the First Conference on Auditory Perceptual Problems and Remediation, Akron, Ohio, University of Akron Press, 1972, p. 12.

exercises in this chapter are intended to improve connected language facility.

DISCRIMINATION FOR PHRASES AND SENTENCES

Step I. Choose a number of pictures to which a simple, appropriate caption may be added. Present the written phrase or sentence with each picture. Give the phrase or sentence orally several times. Be sure to articulate slowly and precisely. Gradually the connected language may be presented more rapidly. Language should be verbalized at a comfortable level of loudness. Use only two or three phrases or sentences at first sittings, then gradually increase the number.

Step II. The speaker should obscure his lips and give ONE phrase or sentence. The listener should identify the appropriate picture by pointing or by repeating the phrase or sentence. The phrases or sentences should be of differing length in early lessons, in order to provide greater contrast for the listener. As he gains skill, the connected language presentations may be more nearly the same length.

Examples of graduations of difficulty:

1. The horse ran
   Three little ducks said "Quack, quack, quack"!
2. The horse ran
   The cow jumped over the moon.
3. The cow jumped over the moon.
   Mother baked a cake.
4. The cow jumped over the moon.
   Mother baked a chocolate cake.
5. The horse ran.
   Father is a man.

Step III. Gradually reduce the level of loudness to force the listener to *develop attending ability.*

Step IV. Introduce a gradually increasing time lapse to *develop auditory memory span.*

Step V. Gradually *increase the number* of phrases or sentences at a given sitting to five or more. Increase the level of loudness to a comfortable listening level each time the number is increased. Reduce the volume, when the listener can fairly consistently identify the phrases or sentences.

Step VI. Introduce a gradually increasing time lapse to *develop auditory memory span.*

Step VII. Repeat the above exercises from various points in the room. The listener should be assisted to demonstrate *localization* ability by correctly identifying the direction from which the signal originated.

Station two or three persons at various points in the room. They should alternate, giving a phrase or sentence. The listener should point to the direction from which the signal came, or they may identify the speaker by name. This *develops discrimination for localization of sound.* This should be presented at a loud level of volume, then gradually reduced. Remember, it will be necessary to use binaural hearing aids for this exercise. If this is not possible, use NO AMPLIFICATION AT ALL. Monaural amplification will not *localize* the sound for the listener.

Step VIII. Give two phrases or sentences from among a choice of three. The listener must now *identify them in the correct sequence.* This should be at a comfortable listening level at first, then with gradually decreased volume as the listener's skill permits.

Step IX. Gradually increase the number to five. Increase the number given in sequence if the listener can handle this much material. Gradually reduce the volume as the listener gains skill.

Step X. Move a short distance from the listener and repeat the above exercises in this part. This forces *projected listening.* Gradually increase the distance. This is a psychological factor as well as a physical space factor.

Step XI. Develop *discrimination for pitch* using phrases and sentences. The listener must identify pitch by some pre-arranged method such as pointing upward, downward, saying "high" and "low." The speaker should maintain either high or low voice throughout, at first. Then as the listener gains skill, he can alternate between high and low pitch within a given sentence. The volume should be comfortably loud.

Step XII. Gradually reduce the volume for the above exercise.

Step XIII. Develop discrimination for loudness and softness, using phrases and sentences. Follow the same procedures as those used in developing discrimination for loudness and softness using vowels, syllables, and words.

Step XIV. A. Show a picture depicting a given situation. Orient the listener that the connected speech will be based on this given situation, such as objects found on the dinner table. The sentence should be well within the listener's vocabulary range, or the exercise will be useless. It may be well to use review vocabulary prior to presentation of this exercise. Give the sentences slowly and under comfortably loud amplification. Give an example or two, with your lips uncovered, so the listener can profit from lip-reading as well as auditory training. Now the speaker should repeat the sentences or phrases with his lips covered. The listener may point to the appropriate picture, repeat the phrase, or write what he hears, in full, or that part which he is able to discern. Examples for dinner table situation picture:

This is a table.
There are four plates on the table.
There is a blue tablecloth on the table.
There are three cups on the table.
There is one glass of milk on the table.
There is a napkin beside each plate.

B. Now, gradually reduce the volume, if possible, for this exercise.

Step XV. Assist the listener to develop *discrimination for Rhythm of Speech* phrases and sentences in the same manner in which you developed rhythm in vowels, syllables, and words.

Step XVI. Develop *discrimination for inflection* of sounds using phrases and sentences in the same manner in which you developed discrimination for inflection of vowels, syllables, and words.

Step XVII. Repeat all exercises in this part with the added dimension of background sound which the listener must learn to "tune out."

For the Hearing Impaired:

Repeat all lessons in this section with gradually reduced levels of loudness. At a comfortable level of loudness for the presentation, introduce soft background sound into the listening situation. Gradually increase the level of background to the extent that the listener can tolerate it and still attend to the lesson content.

DISCRIMINATION FOR SPONTANEOUS CONNECTED SPEECH

Step I. Depending on the age, degree of hearing loss, attention span, and other pertinent factors, the listener may be unable to fully participate in this facet of auditory training. Language should be within the capability of the listener. There is no reason, however, why new vocabulary should not be developed in these lessons, (this should be introduced under amplification).

A. Do some review work without pictures or written materials as clues. The speaker should, however, orient the listener that the language will be based upon a given situation, such as a grocery store, a bridge party, etc.

B. The speaker will present the connected language. The listener will repeat the words or phrases which he is able to discern, or he may paraphrase the entire situation depending upon the listener's skill. The volume should be comfortably loud, at first, then gradually reduced.

Step II. Repeat the above exercises, but *allow a time lapse* between giving the material and asking the listener to identify it, in order to *develop* auditory memory span.

Step III. The speaker should move gradually farther away from the microphone and repeat exercises in this part, to develop *projected listening abilities.* The speaker's lips should be obscured.

Step IV. Repeat the exercises in this part, using pre-recorded materials, first under the auditory training unit, then using the listener's own hearing aid. Volume should be comfortably loud at first, then gradually reduced.

Step V. Develop localization of sound for connected language in the same manner in which you developed this dimension using syllables and words.

Step VI. Develop *discrimination for pitch, using connected language.* Follow the same procedures as those used in developing syllables and words. Gradually reduce the volume.

Step VII. Develop *discrimination for loudness and softness* using connected language. This should be easier for the listener at this stage of his auditory training. Always instruct the listener what he is listening for!

Step VIII. Develop *discrimination for Rhythm of connected language.* Approach it in the same manner as you did for syllables and words.

Step IX. Introduce one or two new words into known situational material. See if the listener can identify the words and obtain meaning from the context of the language. Ask simple questions about material covered.

Step X. Develop *discrimination for inflection of connected language.* Be sure the listener understands what he is listening for, and how to respond.

Step XI. Repeat all exercises in this part, with slight background sound. Gradually increase it as the listener gains skill in discrimination.

Step XII. Present *two* situational pictures. Instruct the listener that he is to listen closely while you give the two sentences, under comfortably loud amplification, in a given order. As soon as the listener has received enough clues to make identification of the picture under discussion, he may do so. Gradually reduce volume. Repeat.

Step XIII. Gradually increase the number of situational pictures for the above exercise.

Step XIV. Repeat all exercises in this part *against slight background sound.* Gradually increase the volume of the background sound as the listener gains skill. Decrease the volume of your voice if possible.

Step XV. Repeat the part dealing with vowels and work through the workbook. This time, allow the listener or listeners, to do the speaking. Always be ready to assist or supplement when necessary, for understanding.

For the Hearing Impaired.

Repeat exercises in this part using the listener's *own hearing aid* as the means of amplification. Gradually reduce volume if possible.

SUGGESTIONS FOR UNSTRUCTURED EXERCISES IN AUDITORY PERCEPTUAL TRAINING

Step I. Review any or all materials in this manual. Present materials in any order. This may be either loud or soft in volume. You must, however, instruct the listener how to respond.

Step II. Vary the methods and procedures such as at greater distances, in sequence, at varying volumes, identifying rhythm, inflection, pitch, and other factors.

Step III. Dictate all kinds of materials, ranging from syllables, counting, words, phrases, sentences, or connected language. The listener should be instructed how to respond. You may have him point, repeat, or write to identify.

Step IV. Repeat any or all exercises with reduced volume.

Step V. Repeat any or all exercises using only the listener's own hearing aid.

Step VI. Repeat any or all exercises, introducing background sound of gradually increasing intensity.

Step VII. Repeat any or all exercises without amplification. This may be very difficult and may require a "practice run" before it will be successful.

Step VIII. Using amplification, engage the listener or listeners in conversation. Give sentences (from review material if you wish, then from new material), which can be answered "yes" or "no." Give "True" or "False" sentences.

Step IX. Use Auditory Training procedures to teach all subject matter if it is to be used in the classroom situation. It may be used profitably to introduce new materials to persons with impaired hearing at all ages and in all situations.

Perhaps one of the most useful results of such a program of auditory training will be found to be the increased ability to attend and concentrate. This must be carried over into general life situations. The therapist or teacher will advise many ways of accomplishing this carry over aspect of Auditory Training.

The reader's attention is again directed to the importance of developing simple, concise lessons each of which should include a checklist of listener responses. This will avoid much confusion and frustration for both the teacher and listener.

The teacher may refer to selected sample lesson plans in the text of this book and to those in the appendix. However, she should be strongly encouraged to develop her own lessons based upon the sequential outline in this book, as quickly as possible.

Teachers of children with auditory perceptual disabilities may feel isolated in their attempts to work with these problems. Often they will feel that there is no one with whom they can discuss the case, the techniques, and the progress. This need not be the case. In any school system there are several sources with whom the teacher or therapist can consult. Teachers and therapists can consult with each other. They can consult with their supervisors. They should discuss their efforts freely with the school psychologist, the teacher of special children, with Instructional Materials Directors. Audio-Visual Aids Consultants will be highly interested in providing suggestions for materials to implement the program. Departments of Speech and Hearing Therapy or Special Education in nearby universities can be contacted for ideas. The author would be willing to offer suggestions to teachers who have very specific questions which she has been unable to satisfy.

APPENDIX I[1]

TWENTY-SIX BEGINNING AUDITORY TRAINING LESSONS

Lesson One

Purpose: To help the children develop an awareness of gross sound in the environment.

Help the children in your class understand where sound comes from. Sound comes from objects in our environment that are rubbed together, struck, or moved quickly in the air in such a way that they vibrate. The cricket rubs his hind legs together to make sound. Rub two sandblocks together to illustrate. Allow several children to rub the sandblocks together. Ask the children to name things in the room that make noise. Make a list of the things that make sound outside the room. (Have the children listen for them.)

Lesson Two

Purpose: To help the children develop an awareness of gross sound in the environment (cowbell) and act upon what they hear.

Review the names of objects that make sound in and outside the room. Help the children understand that certain sounds make us do things. When we are riding our bicycles and we hear a car horn, we know we must be careful and move to the side of the road. When we hear a siren we know that a fire truck, ambulance,

[1] Richard G. Dickerhoof, Educational Audiologist, Stark County Department of Education, Louisville, Ohio.

or police car is coming and we should be careful not to get in their way. Have the children name other sounds that make us do special things. (Firebell, doorbell, recess bell, etc., are good examples.) Explain that the class is going to play a game. Have the children put their heads down. No peeking. When the *cowbell* is sounded have the children raise their heads. Repeat the exercise until each child can accurately respond when the cowbell is sounded.

Lesson Three

Purpose: To help the children develop an awareness of gross environmental sound in the form of music.

Review the activity from lesson two. Continue until the children can accurately respond to the cowbell. Once they have mastered this activity have the children stand in a circle. Place a record on the record player. (Use children's music if possible.) When the music is heard, the children are to walk in a circle. Stop the music at different times. Instruct the children to stop walking when the music stops. *The music should be played at a comfortable listening level.* Continue until the children can accurately respond to the music.

Lesson Four

Purpose: To help the children develop an awareness of gross environmental sound in the form of music.

Review the activity from lesson three. Repeat the exercise. This time have the children either march or skip around the circle in time with the music. Try to help those children having difficulty by having a better listener march next to them. Attempt to refine the children's abilities to listen by gradually decreasing the volume of the music. Continue with this exercise until all children can accurately respond to the music.

Lesson Five

Purpose: To help the children discriminate between two noise makers when only one is sounded.

Review lesson four if the children are still having difficulty. If the children appear to have grasped the concept and are responding correctly, place two noise makers on a tray in the front of the room. (These instruments should sound very different. Suggested noise makers to be used in this section on gross sound discrimination are: drum, cowbell, sandblocks, triangle and whistle.) Using the drum and cowbell, name the instruments for the children and sound each. Let some of the children come to the front and sound the instruments. Have the children put their heads down. No one should be looking. Sound one of the instruments, return it to its original position and then instruct the children to raise their heads and identify the instrument. If they are correct, praise them. If they are incorrect, sound the instrument three times for them: (1) with them watching, (2) with their heads down listening and (3) with the children watching. (This type of teacher response should be used throughout the entire program when evaluating the response of the class or an individual child.)

Lesson Six

Purpose: To help the children discriminate between two and three instruments when one is sounded.

Review the activities from lesson five. Continue the exercise until the children can consistently discriminate between the two noise makers when only one is sounded. When the children can accurately identify the instrument sounded, add a third noise maker—the sandblocks. Name the instrument for the child and sound it for them. Repeat the exercise. Sound only one instrument while the children's heads are down. Vary the instruments among the three possible choices. Return the instrument to its original position and then ask the children to identify the instrument. Reward or correct in the manner suggested earlier. Practice the activity by having individual children identify the sounded instrument. Help the children respond correctly through repeated listenings.

Lesson Seven

Purpose: To help the children discriminate between three and four instruments when only one is sounded.

Review the activities from lesson six. Continue the exercise until the children can consistently discriminate between three instruments when only one is sounded. When the children can accurately identify the sounded instrument under these conditions, add a fourth instrument—the triangle. Name the instrument for the children and sound it for them. Sound the other instruments so that the class can hear the difference. Repeat the exercise. Sound only one instrument while the children's heads are down. Return it to its original position and then ask the children to identify the noise maker. Vary the instrument sounded among the four possible choices. Reward or correct the children in the manner suggested earlier. Practice the activity by playing a game. Divide the class into four teams and assign one instrument to each team. When an instrument is sounded, the team to which that instrument was assigned must respond. If an error is made, the team making the error gets one point. Play to five; the team with the *least* number of points wins.

Lesson Eight

Purpose: To help the children discriminate between four and five noise makers when only one is sounded.

Review the activities from lesson seven. Continue the exercise until the children can consistently discriminate between the four noise makers when only one is sounded. When the children can accurately identify the sounded instrument, add a fifth instrument—the whistle. Name the instrument for the children and sound it for them. Sound the other instruments so that the class can hear the difference. Repeat the exercise. Sound only one instrument while the children's heads are down. Return the instrument to its original position and then ask the children to identify the sounded instrument. Vary the instrument sounded among the five possible choices. Reward or correct the children in the manner suggested earlier. Practice until the children can consistently discriminate between the five noise makers when only one is sounded.

Lesson Nine (Test Number One)

Purpose: To evaluate individual abilities to discriminate between two, three, four, and five noise makers when only one is sounded.

Each child will receive the following form. The test will be a repetition of the previous exercises. For exercise one, only two

TEST FORM # 1

Section I: Drum and Bell

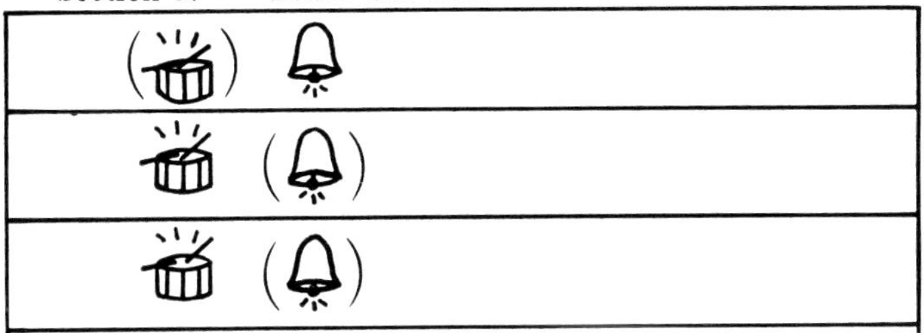

Section II: Drum, Bell, and Sandblocks

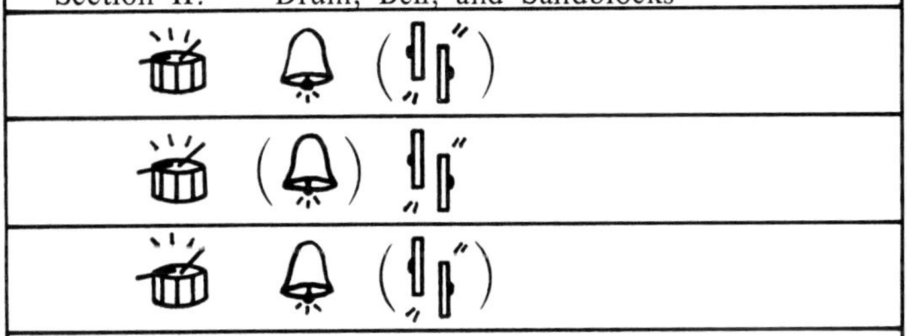

Section III: Drum, Bell, Sandblocks, and Triangle

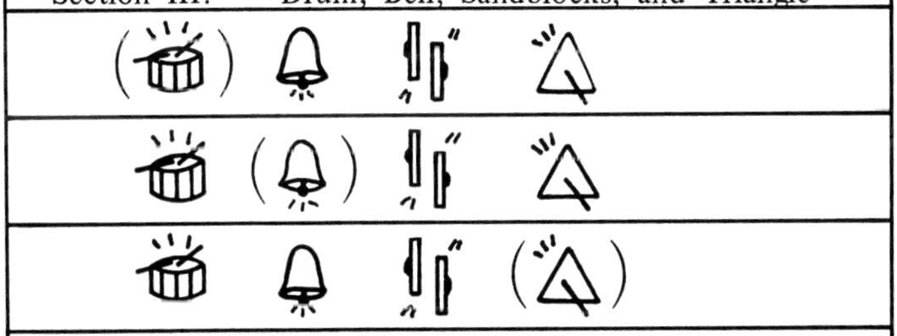

Section IV: Drum, Bell, Sandblocks, Triangle, and Whistle

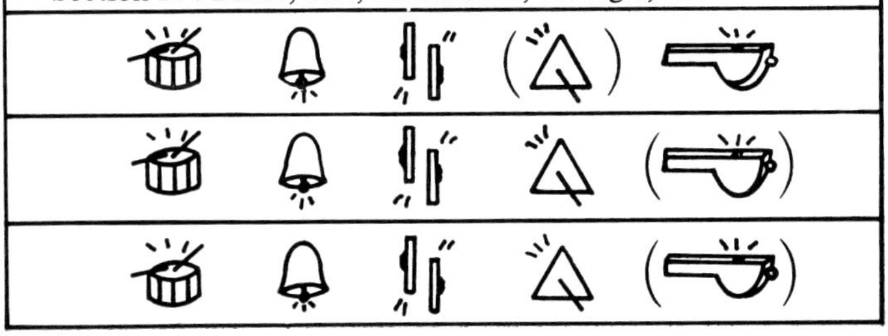

instruments will be placed in front of the room. The children will put their heads on their desks while the teacher sounds one instrument. The children will circle, underline or cross-out the instrument sounded. Each child should be able to accurately identify each instrument sounded. Grade their efforts. More practice may be needed. If so, repeat the lessons where extra help is needed.

Lesson Ten

Purpose: To help the children discriminate between five noise makers when only one is sounded under conditions of reduced volume.

Assuming the children can accurately discriminate between the five noise makers when only one is sounded and have performed adequately on Test #1, continue with the following exercise. Make a tape recording of a lesson similar to the one presented in lesson eight. Play the sound of one instrument; stop; ask the class then to identify the instrument heard. Play several instruments and check the children's discrimination. When the children can accurately identify the noise maker heard on the tape recorder, gradually reduce the volume of the recording. Play several more of the noise makers on the tape recorder. Reward or correct the children in the manner described earlier. Check the children's discrimination. *Do not reduce the volume of the tape recorder until they can consistently make correct identifications at this level.* Attempt to lower the volume through repetitions of the exercise. *Note the volume level on the tape recorder at which the children can correctly identify the instruments only 50% of the time. Save* this recording for later use.

Lesson Eleven

Purpose: To help the children discriminate between five noise makers when only one is sounded under the condition of reduced volume.

Repeat the exercise from lesson ten. Attempt to help the child respond correctly at volume levels lower than those experienced in lesson ten. *Remember to reduce the volume only when the children can correctly identify the instruments presented at that level. Note the lowest volume at which the children can consistently identify the instrument sounded. This level will be important in* future lessons.

Lesson Twelve

Purpose: To help the children discriminate between five noise makers when only one is sounded under conditions of increased background noise.

Repeat the activity from lesson ten. Continue the exercise if the children appear to have difficulty responding to volume levels which are not reasonably soft. If the class appears to accurately respond at extremely soft intensity levels, continue with the following exercise. Using the five noise makers (not tape recorded, but live), repeat the exercise. Sound one instrument while the children's heads are down. Return it to its original position and then ask the children to identify the instrument sounded. Reward or correct the children in the manner suggested earlier. Gradually introduce a background noise: children's music played on a record player. If the children can accurately identify the instrument sounded under these conditions, gradually increase the volume of the background noise. (Be careful not to sound the instruments any louder than you did initially.) Each time the volume of the background noise is increased, check the children's discrimination. *Do not increase the volume of the background noise until the children can consistently make accurate identifications at that volume level. Note this volume setting on the record player. It will be important in later lessons.*

Lesson Thirteen

Purpose: To help the children discriminate between five noise makers when only one is sounded under the condition of increased background noise.

Repeat the exercise from lesson twelve. Begin the exercise using background noise set to the maximum volume at which the children can consistently make accurate identifications of the noise maker sounded. Sound several of the instruments, each time checking the children's discrimination. Reward or correct the children in the manner described earlier. Increase the volume of the background noise only if the children can accurately identify the instruments sounded at that volume level. (Remember not to sound the instruments any louder than you did when the background noise was not present.) Attempt to help the children respond consistently at background noise volumes louder than they experienced in lesson twelve. *Note the maximum volume level of the background noise at which the children can consistently identify the instruments sounded. This volume level will* be important in future lessons.

Lesson Fourteen

Purpose: To evaluate individual abilities to discriminate between five noise makers when only one is sounded under the conditions of (a) reduced volume, and (b) increased background noise.

The following test should be given in two parts. However, the children's answer sheet will be the same for each part.

Part one will consist of listening under conditions of reduced volume. Part two will consist of listening under conditions of increased background noise. The tests will be repetitions of the previous exercises. For each test, three instruments will be sounded at each level of presentations. (1) *Reduced volume:* three instruments will be sounded at that level before reducing the volume. (2) *Background noise:* three instruments will be sounded at each level before the background noise is increased. Volume for Part I should be the level at which the class could accurately identify the instruments during the teaching sessions. Likewise, the highest level of background noise should be the highest volume at which the children could accurately identify the instruments sounded during the teaching session. Following is an example of an answer sheet that may be used.

Children are to mark their answer. Grade their efforts. Repeat those exercises on which the children need special help.

TEST FORM # 2

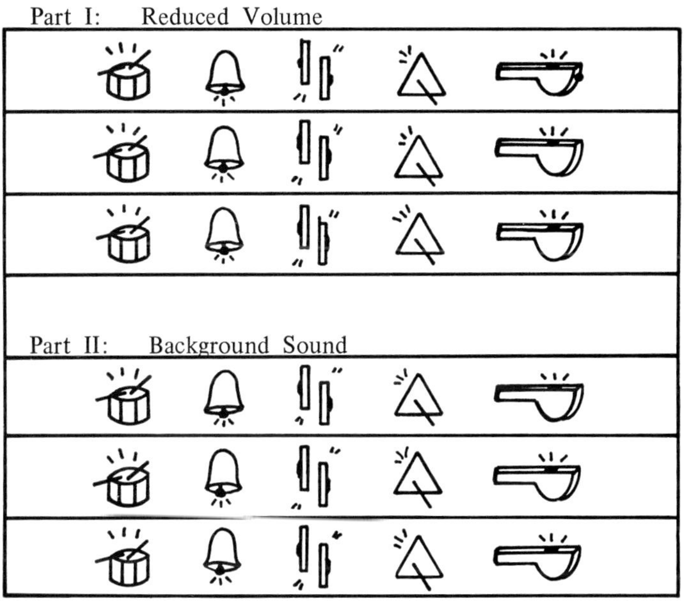

Lesson Fifteen

Purpose: To help develop auditory memory for the discrimination between two noise makers when only one is sounded.

If the children can accurately discriminate between five musical instruments when only one is sounded under conditions of reduced volume and increased background noise, continue with the following: Review the discrimination of two noise makers when only one is sounded. If the children can accurately identify the instrument sounded, repeat the exercise and introduce a time lapse between the time the instrument is sounded and the time the children identify the instrument. Start with a count of two. Sound the instrument. Return it to its original position. Count to two slowly, and then ask the children to identify the instrument sounded. Continue with the exercise until the children can accurately identify the instruments sounded.

Lesson Sixteen

Purpose: To help develop auditory memory for the discrimination between two noise makers when only one is sounded.

Repeat the activities from lesson fifteen. If the children can accurately identify the instrument after a two-count time delay, introduce a four-count time lapse. Count to four slowly and ask the children to identify the instrument. Repeat this exercise several times. Check the children's discrimination. If the class can accurately identify the instrument sounded after a count of four, increase the time lapse to six counts. Using the same procedures, attempt to help the children accurately identify the sounded instrument at this time-lapse level.

Lesson Seventeen

Purpose: To help develop auditory memory for the discrimination between two noise makers when only one is sounded.

Repeat the exercises from lesson sixteen. Help the children accurately identify the instrument after a time lapse of four and six counts. Increase the time lapse to eight counts. Use the same procedures. Repeat the exercise several times. Check the children's discrimination. If the children can accurately identify the sounded instrument after a slow count of eight, increase the time lapse to ten. *Do not attempt to increase the time lapse until the children can accurately identify the instruments at the eight-count level.* Repeat the exercise using the same procedures until the children can adequately discriminate at the ten-count level.

Lesson Eighteen

Purpose: To develop auditory memory for the discrimination between three instruments when only one is sounded.

Repeat the exercises from lesson seventeen. When the children can accurately discriminate between two noise makers when only one is sounded under the condition of a ten-count time lapse, increase the number of possible choices to three: the drum, cowbell and sandblocks. Use a time lapse of ten counts and continue using the procedures described earlier. Count to ten slowly and ask the children to identify the instrument. Help the children respond consistently by repeating the exercise several times. Continue until the children can accurately discriminate between three noise makers when only one is sounded under the condition of a ten-count time lapse.

Lesson Nineteen

Purpose: To develop auditory memory for the discrimination between four noise makers when only one is sounded.

Repeat the exercise from lesson eighteen. Assist the children to respond correctly in discriminating between three noise makers when only one is sounded. Repeat the exercise. Add a fourth instrument; the triangle. Use a time lapse of ten counts. Sound the instrument. Return it to its original position. Count to ten and then ask the children to identify the sounded instrument. Repeat the exercise until the children can consistently identify the instrument from among four choices after a count of ten.

Lesson Twenty

Purpose: To develop auditory memory for the discrimination of five noise makers when only one is sounded.

Repeat the exercise from lesson nineteen. If the children can accurately identify the sounded instrument after a time lapse of ten counts when four possible choices could be made, repeat the exercise adding a fifth instrument, the whistle. Use a count of ten. Sound one of the instruments. Return it to its original position. Count to ten slowly and then ask the children to identify the sounded instrument. Continue the exercise until the children can consistently make accurate identification of the instrument sounded after a count of ten, when five possible choices could be made.

Lesson Twenty-One

Purpose: To evaluate individual abilities of auditory memory for the discrimination of up to five noise makers when only one is sounded.

The following evaluation will take the exact form of Test #1, presented in lesson nine. The test form from that day may also be used. A time lapse of ten counts will be used throughout the examination. Set #1 will have two instruments in the children's view. While the children's heads are down, one instrument will be sounded. Return it to its original position. Count to ten slowly and then ask the children to identify the instrument by marking their paper. Continue in this manner through set #4 where five instruments are used. Continue using the ten-count time delay. Grade the children's efforts. All should be able to consistently identify the sounded instrument after a count of ten when five possible choices could be made. If further practice is needed in certain areas, repeat the exercises dealing with these levels until accurate identifications can be made.

Lesson Twenty-Two

Purpose: To develop auditory memory for the discrimination of five noise makers when only one is sounded under the condition of reduced volume.

If all the children can consistently make accurate identifications of the five noise makers after a ten-count lapse, introduce the following exercise: Use the tape recording of five noise makers that was employed during lesson ten. Remember to play the sound of only one instrument at a time. *Use the ten-count time lapse presented in the earlier lessons.* Play the sound of one instrument. Count to ten slowly and then ask the children to identify the instrument heard. Reward or correct the children in the manner prescribed earlier. Check the children's discrimination. Begin to reduce the volume of the tape recorder. Sound several more of the instruments; check the children's discrimination. Lower the volume of the recording. *Do not reduce the volume of the tape recorder until the class can consistently make correct instrument identifications at that level.* Attempt to lower the volume through repetitions of the exercise. The goal is to lower the volume to that volume at which the children could consistently make accurate instrument identifications of five noise makers when only one was sounded.

Lesson Twenty-Three

Purpose: To develop auditory memory for the discrimination of five noise makers when only one is sounded under the condition of reduced volume.

Repeat the exercise from lesson twenty-two. Help the children to respond consistently at lower and lower volume levels. Attempt to lower the volume of the tape recorder below the volume level at which they could consistently identify five noise makers when only one is sounded. Continue to use a ten-count time lapse. *Note the volume level on the tape recorder at which they could consistently identify five noise makers after a ten count time lapse, when only one was sounded under the condition of reduced volume. This level will be important in future lessons.*

Lesson Twenty-Four

Purpose: To develop auditory memory for the discrimination of five noise makers when only one is sounded, under the condition of increased background noise.

If all the children can consistently make accurate identifications of the five noise makers after a ten-count time lapse and when presented at reduced volume levels, continue with the following exercise: Using the five noise makers, repeat the exercise used in lesson twenty. A ten-count time lapse will be used. Sound several of the instruments waiting the prescribed amount of time before asking for their choice. When the children can accurately identify the instruments sounded, gradually introduce a background noise (the children's music used before). Sound several of the instruments under this condition. Check the children's discrimination. Increase the volume of the background noise when the children can consistently make accurate identifications of the instruments sounded. Continue increasing the volume of the background noise. The goal is to increase the volume of the background noise to the volume at which the children could accurately identify the noise makers in lesson thirteen. Repeat the exercise at this volume level until all the children can accurately identify the sounded noise maker.

Lesson Twenty-Five

Purpose: To develop auditory memory for the discrimination between five noise makers when only one is sounded under the conditions of increased background noise.

Repeat the exercises from lesson twenty-five. Attempt to increase the background noise level beyond that achieved in lesson thirteen. Sound several instruments, waiting the prescribed amount of time. Check the children's discrimination. *Do not attempt to increase the volume of the background noise until the children can consistently make accurate identifications of the sounded instruments at that volume level. Note the highest volume on the record player at which the class can consistently make accurate discriminations between five noise makers, after a ten-count time lapse when only one is sounded under the condition of increased background noise. This volume level will be important in future lessons.*

Lesson Twenty-Six

Purpose: To evaluate individual abilities in auditory memory for discrimination between five noise makers when only one is sounded under the conditions of (a) reduced volume, and (b) increased background noise.

As in lesson fourteen, the following evaluation will be performed in two parts: (a) reduced volume of instruments, and (b) increased background noise. *This time a ten-count time lapse will be inserted before the children mark their papers.* The test procedures will be similar to those used in lesson fourteen. Three instrument presentations will be made at each volume level: I. volume level of the presentation, II. volume level of background noise.

The steps used in either lowering the volume of the presentations or increasing the volume of the background noise should be similar to those used in the teaching sessions. The lowest volume reduction in part one of this evaluation is the setting at which the class could accurately identify the instruments in lesson twenty-three. Likewise, the *highest* volume level to which the background noise should be raised is the highest level at which the children could accurately identify the sounded instrument (lesson twenty-five). At least four different volume levels should be used during each section of the evaluation. The test form will be the same as the one used in lesson fourteen.

The children will mark their answer on the paper. Grade their efforts. All the children should be able to accurately identify the sounded instruments at their lowest level of presentation and at the highest amount of background noise.

APPENDIX II[1]

MATERIALS FOR REMEDIATING SENSORY/PERCEPTUAL PROBLEMS

Introduction

This listing is intended as a representative sampling of commercial materials available for the remediation of sensory-perceptual problems. It should not be considered a comprehensive survey.

Materials are categorized by their apparent primary use. However, many materials could be used interchangeably. Other items, such as ropes, balls, bells, etc. which might be profitably employed by creative teachers are not listed but should certainly be considered. In some areas, no specific commercial material has been developed and the listing of related materials has been eliminated.

Each section begins with (A) an operational definition and (B) an illustration of basic learning abilities for use in developing specific educational programs. Headings and definitions were partially excerpted and adapted from the Remediation of *Learning Disabilities* by Robert E. Vallett. Addresses of publishers are listed in the last section of this contribution.

Similar materials may be viewed at the Special Education Instructional Resource Center serving your area and may be borrowed by teachers of handicapped children for evaluation in classrooms.

[1] Eunice Shonk, Coordinator, Instructional Resource Center, Louisville, Ohio.

MATERIALS FOR REMEDIATING AUDITORY-SENSORY/PERCEPTUAL PROBLEMS

I. *Auditory Acuity*

A. The ability to receive auditory stimuli.
B. Pupil responds functionally to watch tick, hidden sound toys, etc. Pupil has no significant decibel loss.

Related Materials

Bowmar Pub. Co.	*Child's World of Sound,* record.
Concept Records.	*Basic Training in Auditory Perception:* Vol. 3, record.
Creative Playthings.	*Sound Cylinders,* device.
DLM	*Buzzer Board & Pattern Cards,* device.
	Step Bells, device.
Electronics Corp.	*Echorder Automatic Speech & Language Training Aid,* Equip.
Electronics, Inc.	*Phonic Mirror,* equipment.

II. *Auditory Reception*

A. Ability to understand that sounds have meaning and to understand sounds in spoken words.
B. Pupil can respond to oral questions as "Do birds fly?"

Related Materials

Bowmar.	*Listening Time,* record.
Children's Music Center.	*Learning to Listen,* record.
Educational Activities.	*Who Said it?* record and cards.
Educational Record Sales.	*Sounds for Young Readers,* record.
Speech & Language Materials.	*Speech Lingo Game,* game.
Word Making Productions.	*Word Making Cards.*

III. *Auditory Discrimination* *

A. Ability to recognize and differentiate sounds in various situations.*

B. Pupil can indicate by gesture or words differentiation between sounds.

Related Materials

1. Child recognizes & differentiates gross sounds.

Classroom mtls.	*Listening Skills for Pre-Readers,* record.
Concept Records.	*Training in Sound Discrimination,* Vol. 1, record.
DLM	*Auditory Training Familiar Sounds,* tape.
	Auditory Perception Training: Discrimination, fs & tape.
Educational Innovations.	*Auditory Discrimination,* tape & worksheets.
	Sound of Things I see, tape & worksheets.
	Listening Experiences, tape & worksheets.
Eye Gate.	*Our Wonderful World,* f.s. and records.
Milliken.	*It's Fun to Listen,* record, spirit masters.
Radiant Corp.	*Follow through with Sounds: Indoor, Outdoor,* tapes, transparencies.
	Follow through with Sounds: Classroom, Rhythmn, tapes, transparencies.
Scott Foresman.	*Sounds I can Hear,* record and cards.
3M.	*Sounds at Home,* tape and worksheets.
H. Wilson Corp.	*World of Sound,* record.

* Materials should be varied or developed to allow practice involving variations in pitch, intensity, duration, volume, tempo.

2. Child recognizes & differentiates alphabet sounds in isolation.

McGraw Hill.	*Stories for Listening*, records.
Phonovisual Products.	*Phonovisual Charts*, chart.
Teaching Resources.	*Auditory Discrimination in Depth*, tapes & worksheets.

3. Child recognizes & differentiates alphabet sounds in words.

Bowmar.	*Singing Sounds*, record.
Children's Music Center.	*Listen & Learn*, record.
Concept Records.	*Introduction to Speech Elements*, record.
Educational Activities.	*Listen & Learn with Sparky*, workbook, record.
Follett.	*Junior Listen-Hear Program*, books, record.
Houghton-Mifflin.	*Listen & Do*, records and worksheets.
Ideal.	*Animated Key Cards*, cards.
	Magic Cards, laminated cards.
	Vowels Structured Reading Tapes, tape & worksheets.
Singer.	*Initial Consonants*, cards.
Speech & Language Materials.	*Auditory Discrimination-Rhyming Words*, cards.
	I-D Puzzles Speech Lingo, game
	Spin-It, game *Peel & Put*, labels.
Univ. of Illinois Press.	*What's Its Name?* book.
Word Making Productions.	*Word Making Cards*, card.
	Snoopy Snake, book.

IV. *Auditory-Motor Coordination*

A. Ability to coordinate body movements in response to auditory input.

B. The pupil will move his body in response to oral commands without gross errors.

Related Materials

Bowmar.	*Songs for Children with Special Needs,* record.
Children's Music Center.	*Get Fit While You Sit,* record.
Educational Activities.	*Listening & Moving Series,* records.
	Chicken Fat, record.
Ginn & Co.	*Brave Hunter,* record.
Rhythm Records.	*Hand Rhythms,* record.
	Pre-School Activities for Young Children, record.

V. *Auditory Figure-Ground*

A. The ability to ignore competing stimuli and attend to a primary signal.
B. Pupil can take direction and respond to verbal stimuli in the presence of competing sounds.

Related Materials

Concept Records.	*Basic Training Vol. 2: Figure Ground Discrimination,* record.
DLM.	*Auditory Perception-Figure Ground,* tapes & worksheets.

VI. *Auditory Position in Space*

A. Ability to localize auditory stimuli in relation to the body.
B. Child can point to the direction from which a sound originates.

VII. *Auditory Memory and Sequencing*

A. Ability to retain & recall auditory information.
B. Pupil can demonstrate recall of sounds, sound patterns, experiences, directions.

Related Materials

1. Recall of single sounds.

Creative Playthings.	*Rhythm Bells,* device.
DLM	*Tok-Bak,* device.
Eye Gate.	*Our Wonderful,* f.s. and records.
Scott Foresman.	*Sounds I can Hear,* records and cards, *Buzzer Board,* device.

2. Recall of sequence of digits, letters, words.

Bowmar.	*Saying the Right Word,* record.
Classroom Mtls. Co.	*Listening Skills for Pre-Readers III,* record.
Milton Bradley.	*Alphabet Poster Cards.*

3. Recall of simple stories, rhymes, experiences.

Bowmar.	*Modern Classics,* record, *Say Along Stories,* record, *Favorite Folktales,* record, *Animals,* record.
Dexter Westbrook.	*Sequent-A-Sets,* cards.
Walt Disney.	*Read Along Kits,* tape/books.
Radiant Corp.	*Expressive Receptive Skills,* tape/books/posters.
Scott Foresman.	*First Talking Storybook,* records and books.

4. Recall of directions.

Educational Innovations, Inc.	*Following Directions,* tape/worksheet.
Houghton Mifflin.	*Listening & Learning,* records/worksheets.
SRA.	*Listening Skills Program,* records.

VIII. *Auditory Association* (Imagery, Generalization, Inference)

A. The ability to use judgment, reasoning and imagery in relation to auditory stimuli.

B. The pupil can verbally classify, generalize, conclude and infer from auditory stimuli (sounds, words, stories, descriptions, etc.)

Related Materials

Bowmar.	*Listening Time Stories,* record, *Best in Children's Literature,* records.
DLM.	*Auditory Perception Training—Imagery,* tapes & worksheets.
Educational Reading Service.	*Junior Library,* books and records.
Field Educational Pub.	*Checkered Flag Series,* f.s.,tapes books.
SRA.	*Listening Skills Program Ia, Ib, Ic, IIa,* records.
Wilson.	*Developing Language Arts Skills,* records.

IX. *Multiple Auditory Sensory/Perceptual Areas*

Bowmar.	*Child's World of Sound,* record.
Classroom Mtls.	*Listening Skills for Pre-Readers,* record.
Teaching Resources.	*A.D.D. Program Auditory Discrimination in Depth.*

MATERIALS FOR REMEDIATING MULTIPLE AREAS OF SENSORY/PERCEPTUAL PROBLEMS

Allied Education Council.	*Shape, Structure & Sequencing,* workbook.
Bowmar.	*The Five Senses,* record, *Sights & Sounds—Series 2,* records.
Concept Records.	*Basic Songs for Exceptional Children, Vol. 1,* record,

Continental Press.	*Thinking Skills*, spirit masters, *Likenesses & Differences*, spirit masters.
Educational Activities.	*Developing Cognitive Skills in Young Learners*, f.s., *Living Basic Skills through Music, Vols. I, II*, record, *Living Basic Skills through Music: Vocabulary*, record.
Field Educational Pub.	*Target Red Series.*
Follett.	*Pictures & Patterns*, workbooks, *Parkinson Program for Special Children*, workbooks, games, devices.
Harper Rowe.	*Learning Readiness System: Classification & Seriation*, transparencies, spirit masters.
Noble & Noble.	*TRY: Experiences for Young Children*, workbooks, devices.
Prentice-Hall.	*Advantage*, workbook.
SRA.	*Learning to Think Series*, workbooks.
Teaching Resources.	*Vanguard School Program*, workbooks.

AUTHOR INDEX

SUBJECT INDEX